THE PSYCHOLOGY OF HALLUCINATIONS

What triggers a hallucination? Can our lifestyles impact the likelihood of auditory or visual hallucinations? Can hallucinations be a part of normal cognition? *The Psychology of Hallucinations* takes readers on a journey through visual and auditory hallucinations—perceptions experienced in the absence of external stimuli yet felt with compelling realism. It explores the ways hallucinations have been embraced throughout history by some cultures whilst also looking at how they have become a subject of scepticism and fear. The book adopts a compassionate look at the clinical and psychiatric implications of hallucinations alongside lifestyle factors such as sleep deprivation and substance use. Whether they represent a doorway to creative revelation, markers of struggle or subjects of philosophical inquiry, hallucinations deserve exploration that is curious, compassionate and clear-eyed. This volume provides just that—a guide for anyone seeking to understand, rather than simply fear, the mysteries at the borders of the mind.

Gabriel Andrade is an Associate Professor at Ajman University, United Arab Emirates. He has previously taught at university level in Venezuela, the Marshall Islands, Aruba and the Cayman Islands. He has written books and articles at the intersection of psychology, ethics, religion and philosophy.

THE PSYCHOLOGY OF EVERYTHING

People are fascinated by psychology, and what makes humans tick. Why do we think and behave the way we do? We've all met arm-chair psychologists claiming to have the answers, and people that ask if psychologists can tell what they're thinking. *The Psychology of Everything* is a series of books which debunk the popular myths and pseudo-science surrounding some of life's biggest questions.

The series explores the hidden psychological factors that drive us, from our subconscious desires and aversions, to our natural social instincts. Absorbing, informative, and always intriguing, each book is written by an expert in the field, examining how research-based knowledge compares with popular wisdom, and showing how psychology can truly enrich our understanding of modern life.

Applying a psychological lens to an array of topics and contemporary concerns - from sex, to fashion, to conspiracy theories - *The Psychology of Everything* will make you look at everything in a new way.

Titles in the series:

The Psychology of Menopause by
Marie Percival

The Psychology of Fashion
Second Edition by Carolyn Mair

The Psychology of the Extreme by
Arie W. Kruglanski and Sophia
Moskalenko

The Psychology of Stress by
Charlotte Mottram,
Alison Woodward,
and Shanti Farrington

The Psychology of Sports Fans by
Aaron CT Smith

The Psychology of Sex 2e by
Meg-John Barker

The Psychology of Money by
Adrian Furnham

The Psychology of Genealogy by
Susan M. Moore

The Psychology of Hallucinations by
Gabriel Andrade

For more information about this series, please visit: www.routledgetextbooks.com/textbooks/thepsychologyofeverything/

THE PSYCHOLOGY OF HALLUCINATIONS

GABRIEL ANDRADE

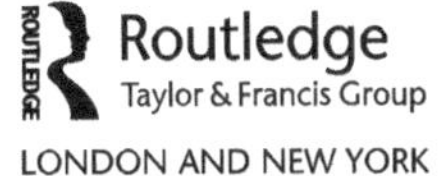

LONDON AND NEW YORK

Designed cover image: Getty Images

First published 2027
by Routledge
4 Park Square, Milton Park, Abingdon, Oxon OX14 4RN

and by Routledge
605 Third Avenue, New York, NY 10158

Routledge is an imprint of the Taylor & Francis Group, an informa business

© 2027 Gabriel Andrade

For Product Safety Concerns and Information please contact our EU representative GPSR@taylorandfrancis.com. Taylor & Francis Verlag GmbH, Kaufingerstraße 24, 80331 München, Germany.

British Library Cataloguing-in-Publication Data
A catalogue record for this book is available from the British Library

ISBN: 9781041328575 (hbk)
ISBN: 9781041328537 (pbk)
ISBN: 9781003784890 (ebk)

DOI: 10.4324/9781003784890

Typeset in Joanna
by KnowledgeWorks Global Ltd.

TABLE OF CONTENTS

INTRODUCTION

In recent years, one of the most frequent concerns of modern life, echoed across newsrooms, social media platforms, and everyday conversation, has been the rise of "fake news." This term has come to signify not only a political or informational problem, but also a deep crisis of epistemology—the question of how we can know what is true, and what counts as reality. The worry about fake news extends beyond journalism or politics; it touches on something fundamental to the human experience: our reliance on perception and representation to access the world.

When a carefully staged video, an image generated by artificial intelligence, or a digitally manipulated recording can circulate globally and be accepted as fact, our traditional confidence in sensory evidence begins to erode. Events that never happened are experienced as vividly as those that did. A photo of a politician in a fabricated scandal, viewed by millions, may provoke anger, emotion, or belief even after being proven false. The phenomenon of "deepfakes"—AI-created images or videos indistinguishable from real footage—makes this even more acute (Karnouskos, 2020). Here, the entire notion of authenticity collapses under the weight of simulation.

DOI: 10.4324/9781003784890-1

These developments invite us to reconsider not only the reliability of our media environment, but also the reliability of our minds. Seeing something—whether online or before our eyes—no longer guarantees that it exists in the form we perceive it. The boundaries between reality and representation, perception and imagination, become porous. Within this tension lies a theoretical doorway to the psychology of hallucinations: experiences that feel real, though they arise without a corresponding external object. Before exploring hallucinations themselves, however, it is worth dwelling on the philosophical lineage of this question—one that long predates the digital age.

Jean Baudrillard, the French philosopher and cultural critic, offered perhaps the most striking conceptual framework for understanding this collapse of the real into representation. In works such as *Simulacra and Simulation* (1994), Baudrillard argued that contemporary society had entered a stage where signs no longer refer to underlying realities. Instead, they only refer to other signs in an endless play of simulation. In ancient times, a map was a representation of territory; today, he suggested, the map precedes the territory. The imitation becomes more real than the original—a condition he called hyperreality. In Baudrillard's (1994, p. 22) words, "One must think instead of the media as if they were, in outer orbit, a kind of genetic code that directs the mutation of the real into the hyperreal."

To illustrate, he described Disneyland as the perfect model of the hyperreal. It presents itself as an imaginary world, but this self-conscious fiction masks the fact that the "real" world outside operates under the same logic—constructed, curated, staged. Similarly, in media culture, the distinction between a televised event and its occurrence becomes meaningless. The Gulf War, Baudrillard provocatively wrote, "did not take place"—not because bombs didn't fall or people didn't die, but because the war we experienced was a mediated spectacle, a televised narrative rather than direct experience (Baudrillard, 2009).

In such a world, perception is detached from reality, and the mind becomes increasingly occupied by images, signs, and echoes rather than concrete referents. The line between experiencing and imagining dissolves. This theoretical condition of hyperreality parallels the phenomenological dimension of hallucination: the subject encounters something intensely vivid, emotionally compelling, and experientially immediate, yet untethered from an external cause. Both involve entering a realm where signs or sensations appear autonomous, where the mind projects substance onto nothingness.

Yet these concerns are hardly new. The instability of perception and the uncertainty of reality have been central philosophical preoccupations throughout history. The crisis provoked by "fake news" merely echoes a question that has accompanied human thought since antiquity: how can we know that what we perceive truly corresponds to what is real?

PHILOSOPHERS OF UNCERTAIN WORLDS

One of the earliest and most enduring explorations of this issue lies in Plato's *The Republic*, in the allegory of the cave. Plato asks us to imagine a group of prisoners chained inside a dark cavern, unable to turn their heads. Behind them burns a fire; between the fire and the prisoners is a raised walkway along which unseen figures carry objects. The prisoners see only the flickering shadows of these objects cast upon the wall before them. To them, these shadows are reality, for they have known nothing else. Should one prisoner be freed and ascend to the surface, he would initially be blinded by the sunlight—the true source of illumination—but gradually he would recognise that what he once took for truth was merely illusion (Plato & Lane, 2007).

Plato's image of the cave already gestures toward a problem that will be central to this book: how to distinguish different ways in which experience can depart from what is actually there. The prisoners' shadows are best understood as illusions rather than hallucinations: there is a real fire, real objects, and a real wall, but the sensory information they provide is systematically misleading, so that what is genuinely present is misinterpreted and flattened into two-dimensional silhouettes. By contrast, hallucinations are not distortions of existing stimuli but perception-like experiences arising in the absence of any appropriate external object or event—a voice heard when no one speaks, a figure seen where no one stands, a smell sensed when nothing in the environment could plausibly produce it. The very term "hallucination" comes from the Latin *alucinari* or *hallucinari*, "to wander in the mind" or "to be absent-minded" (Telles-Correia et al., 2015), and contemporary clinical usage preserves this sense of mental wandering: hallucinations are typically defined as vivid, substantial, perception-like experiences that occur without external stimuli, are experienced with the immediacy of real perception, and are not under voluntary control. This distinction between misperceiving what is there (illusion) and perceiving what is not there at all (hallucination) will become crucial as the discussion moves from Plato's cave to the psychological and neuroscientific accounts of hallucinations that follow.

In any case, this parable encapsulates Plato's metaphysics. For him, the world accessible to the senses is not the ultimate reality but a mere shadow of the higher, immutable world of Forms (or Ideas). Every visible object—tree, chair, human face—is merely an imperfect copy of its corresponding ideal Form, which exists in a purely intelligible realm graspable only through reason. Perception deceives; knowledge arises only when the mind ascends beyond the cave of appearances toward the eternal truths.

Across the world, a similar metaphysical dilemma unfolded in ancient China. The philosopher Zhuang Zhou—better known as Zhuangzi—offered one of the most poetic reflections on the uncertainty of perception. In a famous passage, he recounts a dream in which he was a butterfly flitting through the air, entirely content and unaware of his human identity: "Once Zhuang Zhou dreamt he was a butterfly, a butterfly flitting and fluttering around, happy with himself and doing as he pleased. He didn't know he was Zhuang Zhou. Suddenly he woke up and there he was, solid and unmistakable Zhuang Zhou. But he didn't know if he was Zhuang Zhou who had dreamt he was a butterfly, or a butterfly dreaming he was Zhuang Zhou" (Zhuangzi, 2003, p. 44).

This parable captures a radical epistemological scepticism: the distinction between dream and waking life may not be absolute, and the continuity of identity may be illusory. Just as Baudrillard later suggested that society lives within simulations of its own creation, Zhuangzi implied that consciousness moves fluidly between layers of experience that feel equally real. The criterion for reality—whether rooted in external verification or internal conviction—remains elusive.

Zhuangzi's insight also contains a notable psychological resonance. The felt reality of the dream, like that of a hallucination, is not diminished by its lack of external grounding. Within the dream, as within a hallucination, the mind constructs a coherent world complete with sensory richness and emotional meaning. Reality, in such moments, resides not in external validation, but in experience itself.

This motif resurfaced with philosophical precision in the seventeenth century, when René Descartes famously sought to establish a foundation for certain knowledge. Descartes recognised that sensory experience is notoriously unreliable: objects appear smaller at a distance, sticks seem bent in water, and dreams can perfectly imitate waking life. To eliminate all possible doubt, he engaged in a radical thought experiment, imagining the existence of an "evil genius"—a powerful deceiver who manipulates his perceptions and thoughts so that everything he believes to be true might be false.

Suppose, Descartes argued, that such a deceiver could create in me the very sensations and ideas I attribute to the external world. As Descartes (1984, p. 15) famously wrote, "I will suppose therefore that not God, who is supremely good and the source of truth, but rather some malicious demon, had employed his whole energies in deceiving me". How, then, could I distinguish between reality and a perfect illusion? Confronted with this possibility, Descartes could doubt everything—except the fact that he was doubting. From this indubitable act of thinking arose his famous conclusion: *Cogito, ergo sum* ("I think, therefore I am"). Even if an evil genius deceived him about the existence of the physical world, the act of thought itself guaranteed his existence as a thinking subject.

Descartes' philosophical exercise intensified the separation between mind and world, establishing the ground for modern epistemology and cognitive science alike. His hypothetical scenario also resonates strongly with the phenomenology of hallucinations. To experience a hallucination is to live, however momentarily, within a Cartesian nightmare—one's sensory apparatus insists upon the reality of an object that does not exist, and yet the experience feels as incontestable as any genuine perception.

While Descartes ultimately reinstated the external world as real—albeit known imperfectly through reason—another philosopher, George Berkeley, took a more radical route. Writing in the early eighteenth century, Berkeley argued that the very notion of a material world existing independently of perception was incoherent. His idealism rested on a simple but profound proposition: to be is to be perceived (*esse est percipi*) (Berkeley, 1982). Berkeley reasoned that all we ever encounter are ideas and sensations within the mind. When we say that a tree exists, we mean merely that we (or some observer) perceive its colour, shape, texture, and location. The idea of an unperceived tree—something wholly beyond mind—makes no sense, because the very act of conceiving it brings it into perception. Rather than a material reality "out there", Berkeley proposed that the world consists entirely of perceptions sustained by the divine mind, which guarantees the coherence of experience when no human observer is present.

Although Berkeley's intent was theological rather than sceptical, his doctrine attempted to dismantle the assumption that perception points beyond itself. Experience becomes self-contained: all that exists are mental representations. In a peculiar way, this idealist view erases the distinction between normal perception and hallucination. If everything we perceive exists only as an idea within consciousness, then hallucinations differ from ordinary perceptions not in substance but in order or coherence. Both belong to the same ontological realm—the mind's theatre—though one aligns with the divine order and the other does not.

Across these philosophical traditions—from Plato's cave to Baudrillard's hyperreal—the question is not merely epistemological but existential. What is it to be human in a world where perception is uncertain? Each thinker, in his own fashion, arrives at a recognition that reality as experienced is always mediated—by senses, by language, by cultural symbols, or by the mind's own structure.

The worry about "fake news" today carries a secular echo of these metaphysical concerns. When millions interpret a digitally fabricated event as truth, the phenomenon speaks not only to social manipulation but to the fragility of human cognition. Our perceptual systems are not designed to doubt reality; they are tuned to trust their inputs. Once an image or sound satisfies the brain's criteria of coherence and plausibility, it is treated as fact. This same mechanism underlies hallucinations: the mind confers reality upon its own productions when they sufficiently mimic the structure of perception.

In both contexts—the political and the psychological—the challenge is not that we cannot perceive, but that our perceptions are too convincing. Our cognitive architecture inclines us to attribute existence to what feels real, regardless of its source. Philosophers have wrestled with this predicament for millennia; neuroscientists now explore it in terms of prediction errors and perceptual inference (Sedley et al., 2016). Yet the core human problem remains unchanged: how to discern the real from the imagined when both press upon us with equal force.

The terrain of hallucinations thus lies nestled within one of humanity's oldest and most profound inquiries. Fake news troubles our trust in media; hallucinations trouble our trust in the mind. Both compel us to confront the unsettling realisation that reality itself, as we live it, is to a significant degree a construction—an ever-shifting interplay between what is given by the world and what is generated by consciousness.

WHY HALLUCINATIONS MATTER

These philosophical ideas are not just abstract musings—they offer a foundation for psychologists and neuroscientists to study hallucinations as tangible, measurable experiences in human life. Thinkers like Plato, Zhuangzi, Descartes, and Berkeley highlight the tension between appearance and reality; modern psychology takes this further by asking how that divide is represented in the brain and in lived experience, and how frequently it appears in both everyday and clinical contexts. What began as philosophical scepticism about perception has become an empirical question: under what circumstances does the mind create experiences that feel real despite the absence of external stimuli, and how are these experiences shaped by culture, development, and mental health?

Even at a very broad level, hallucinations can be sorted along several dimensions that anticipate the more detailed taxonomies developed later in this book. One basic distinction concerns sensory modality: auditory, visual, tactile, olfactory, gustatory, and somatic hallucinations each have partly distinct neural and phenomenological profiles. Another concerns context and course: transient, non-distressing hallucinations in otherwise healthy individuals; hallucinations embedded in psychotic disorders such as schizophrenia; and hallucinations secondary to neurological or medical conditions (for example, Parkinson's disease, epilepsy, sensory deprivation, or visual loss in Charles Bonnet syndrome). A third axis is the degree of insight: some people recognise their experiences as internally generated, while others attribute them firmly to external agents or forces, often with powerful emotional and behavioural consequences.

Having already distinguished hallucinations from illusions, it helps to lay out the main adjacent phenomena—delusions, ideas of reference, dreams, and altered states of consciousness—before sharpening the differences. In contrast to hallucinations, which are perception-like experiences arising without an appropriate external stimulus, delusions are best understood as beliefs: they are fixed, false convictions held with strong subjective certainty, resistant to counter-argument, and not shared by the person's cultural group, even though they often grow around or incorporate hallucinatory content (for example, a belief about being persecuted by neighbours can be elaborated to explain threatening voices) (Adachi & Akanuma, 2016). Ideas of reference concern the meaning attributed to ordinary events: the person interprets neutral occurrences—a song on the radio, people whispering, a passing car—as carrying a special, often secret message directed specifically at them; in milder forms, this retains some doubt, but with increasing conviction and systematisation it can harden into full delusions of reference (Shives, 2007). Dreams present another neighbouring phenomenon: they are saturated with hallucinatory imagery, yet they occur in sleep, when reality-testing is suspended, and on awakening most people spontaneously reclassify their dream experiences as "not real", whereas waking hallucinations intrude into a state that is ordinarily governed by the expectation of veridical perception and may be taken as genuinely occurring in the here-and-now. Finally, altered states of consciousness—whether induced by substances, sensory deprivation, meditation, trance, or neurological disturbance—primarily involve global shifts in awareness, time perception, and sense of self (Tart, 2000); hallucinations may or may not appear within these states, but altered consciousness is the broader framework, with hallucinations representing one possible content within it rather than its defining feature. Together, these distinctions help to locate hallucinations as a specific kind of experience—percept-like, stimulus-absent, and often reality-endorsed—nested within a wider landscape of how minds can misbelieve, misinterpret, and reconfigure reality.

Empirical work over the past three decades has made it clear that hallucinations are neither rare nor confined to severe mental illness. Large population-based studies suggest that hallucinations of various kinds occur in a substantial minority of people at some point in their lives, often without leading to clinical care. A large systematic review of auditory hallucinations across the lifespan, estimated a mean lifetime prevalence of around 9.6%, with rates of approximately 12–13% in children and adolescents, and 5–6% in adults (Linszen et al., 2022). Epidemiological surveys focused specifically on auditory verbal hallucinations in community samples report lifetime rates between about 5% and 15%, depending on methodology (de Leede-Smith & Barkus, 2013), with one Norwegian postal survey finding that 7.3% of adults reported having heard voices at some point (I. E. Sommer et al., 2010). When hallucinations in all modalities are considered, several large surveys converge on a prevalence range of roughly 6–15% in the general population (Toh et al., 2020), indicating that non-clinical hallucinations are a common, if often hidden, part of human experience.

Age, context, and clinical status modulate these figures in important ways. For example, a large British general population study using consistent measures across the adult lifespan found that the past-year prevalence of hallucinations was about 7% in people aged 16–19 years, declining gradually to around 3% in those aged 70 and older (Yates et al., 2021). In children, a Dutch cohort study of nearly 4,000 participants reported a one-year prevalence of auditory vocal hallucinations of 9% at ages 7–8, though only about 15% of these children experienced substantial suffering or problem behaviour associated with the voices (Bartels-Velthuis et al., 2010). Non-clinical voice hearers in adult samples often report brief, infrequent, and controllable experiences—on average every few days, for a few minutes at a time—with little or no interference in daily life, in stark contrast to the distressing, persistent hallucinations seen in psychotic disorders. Nevertheless, across age groups, the presence of hallucinations in community samples is consistently associated with higher rates of mental disorders, suicidal ideation, and suicide attempts (Linscott & Os, 2013), underlining their significance as risk markers as well as phenomena of intrinsic interest.

There are many reasons why a wide audience should care about hallucinations. Clinically, they are hallmark features of psychotic disorders but also occur in mood disorders, neurodegenerative conditions, sensory impairment, and substance-related states, making them a transdiagnostic phenomenon that transcends traditional diagnostic categories. Even outside formal diagnoses, their presence can indicate elevated risk for mental health difficulties, reduced quality of life, and self-harm, prompting calls for early detection and compassionate, non-stigmatising interventions. Culturally, hallucinations have shaped religious revelations, shamanic and artistic practices, and collective rituals—from ancient vision quests and prophetic voices to modern psychedelic ceremonies—making them central to the study of meaning and belief. Intellectually, they occupy a unique position at the intersection of philosophy, psychology, and neuroscience, illuminating the brain's constructive role in perception, challenging naïve realism about the senses, and revealing how a coherent world-model can both sustain and unravel the lived fabric of experience.

FOLLOWING THE THREADS AHEAD

The chapters that follow take these threads and work them through different levels of explanation, moving from history and culture to brain and clinic, and finally to the intimate texture of lived experience. The opening chapter asks how hallucinations have been understood across times and places—as divine messages, witchcraft, moral failing, artistic inspiration, or signs of madness—and shows how similar experiences can be elevated, tolerated, or pathologised depending on the symbolic and institutional frameworks that surround them. This broader canvas sets the stage for understanding why some people with distressing hallucinations hesitate to seek help, while others actively cultivate such states within religious or aesthetic practices.

From there, the focus turns to mechanisms. One strand examines how the brain constructs perceptual reality and how this constructive process sometimes overshoots its mark. Contemporary models that treat perception as prediction and inference—the brain as hypothesis-tester rather than passive recorder—frame hallucinations as extreme but intelligible outcomes of ordinary processes. The aim of the discussion is not to locate a single "hallucination centre", but to map interacting systems whose balance can be tipped by development, trauma, substances, neurodegeneration, or sensory deprivation.

Subsequent chapters consider the clinical landscapes where hallucinations most often draw professional attention. One landscape is that of psychotic disorders—schizophrenia, schizoaffective disorder, and mood disorders with psychotic features—in which hallucinations are embedded in complex patterns of delusion, disorganisation, and negative symptoms. Another comprises neurological and medical conditions such as Parkinson's disease, epilepsy, dementias, delirium, and profound visual loss, where hallucinations emerge via distinct pathophysiological routes but raise similar questions about insight, risk, and coping. Running through these sections is a concern with trajectories: why experiences that are relatively common and transient in childhood or in the general population become persistent and disabling for some, and how early signs might be recognised without casting every unusual perception as a prodrome.

A separate arc follows hallucinations into the liminal territories of sleep and substances, and then back into subjective meaning and practice. Chapters on hypnagogic and hypnopompic experiences, sleep paralysis, and REM intrusion examine how altered states of arousal and dreaming physiology can flood waking consciousness with images and presences that feel indistinguishable from psychotic hallucinations yet arise through different mechanisms and demand different responses. Parallel discussions of psychedelics and other psychoactive substances show how pharmacological shifts in neuromodulatory systems reshape perception and self-experience, whether in structured ritual and therapeutic settings or in chaotic and coercive ones.

Later chapters turn this understanding toward practice, sketching principles of assessment and intervention—from pharmacological treatment to psychological, trauma-informed, voice-dialogue, peer-led, and community approaches—that seek not only to reduce hallucinations but to transform a person's relationship with them, balancing awareness of risk with an eye to the possibilities opened by insight, support, and culture over time.

Set against the anxieties of fake news and deepfakes, and framed by a long philosophical meditation on the fragility of perception, this journey through hallucinations is not only about a clinical symptom but about a particular vulnerability of human consciousness. To take hallucinations seriously is to acknowledge that the mind is both a receiver and a maker of worlds, that the line between perception and imagination is thin but not arbitrary, and that individual experiences of "seeing what is not there" are entangled with collective struggles over truth, meaning, and authority. The chapters that follow invite the reader to stay with this tension, tracing how brains, cultures, and persons together shape the realities that are inhabited, defended, and sometimes, quite literally, heard and seen.

1

THE HISTORY AND CULTURAL INTERPRETATIONS OF HALLUCINATIONS

In 1429, a teenage peasant from the village of Domrémy was led into the royal castle at Chinon to meet the Dauphin of France, Charles, whose claim to the throne was fragile and widely doubted. Charles, wary of imposture, hid himself among his courtiers in ordinary dress, while another man took a prominent place as if he were king. Joan of Arc—as she would be known— walked past the decoy, crossed the crowded hall and bowed instead to the disguised Dauphin, addressing him as the rightful heir of France. In later retellings, this scene was taken as proof that her guidance could not have come from human advisers alone: An illiterate adolescent, unfamiliar with courtly etiquette, correctly identifying the prince in a hall full of richly dressed nobles because, she said, her voices had directed her (Castor, 2015).

For Joan, those voices had formed the core of her inner world for years before Chinon. She reported first hearing them around the age of 13, accompanied by a great light and a sense of presence she later named as Saint Michael, Saint Catherine and Saint Margaret. The voices did not merely console; they issued clear commands—go to the Dauphin, raise the siege of Orléans, see Charles crowned at Reims—and carried an authority that outweighed family objections,

DOI: 10.4324/9781003784890-2

priestly caution and the obvious risks of war. Her testimony suggests a phenomenology in which auditory experience, occasional visual elements and a powerful feeling of external agency fused into a unified, unquestioned call to action. Whatever their ultimate explanation, these experiences were real enough that she repeatedly risked imprisonment, torture and death rather than deny them.

What makes Joan such a compelling figure for a psychology of hallucinations is not simply that she heard voices, but that those voices were immediately intelligible within the symbolic universe of fifteenth-century France. Saints, angels and heavenly lights occupied familiar places in sermons, miracle stories and devotional art; her experiences drew on a repertoire her contemporaries already recognised as markers of divine communication. Her voices thus arrived pre-labelled as potentially sacred, and when their content aligned with urgent political hopes—liberating besieged cities, restoring a weakened monarchy—they could be received, at least for a time, as signs of God's intervention in history. In many modern contexts, similar perceptual experiences might be cast as symptoms of illness; in Joan's case, the same experiential structure helped mobilise armies and reconfigure national identity.

The drama of her life also shows how precarious that status can be. The same church that would later canonise her first condemned her as a heretic, interrogating her at length about how the voices sounded, where they came from, whether they contradicted doctrine and whether she could be persuaded to renounce their supernatural origin. The boundary between revelation and delusion was negotiated question by question in her trial, as theologians and judges tried to decide whether her inner experiences should be trusted, feared or suppressed. From a psychological perspective, this is an early, public example of a process that recurs across cultures: unusual perceptual experiences are sifted through religious, moral and institutional filters that determine whether they become sources of authority, grounds for punishment or objects of medical concern.

The story of Joan of Arc situates the topic at a point where voice-hearing was neither private symptom nor abstract philosophical puzzle, but a phenomenon that could decide battles and redraw borders. Daniel B. Smith meaningfully writes in his popular book *Muses, Madmen and Prophets: Hearing Voices and the Borders of Sanity*: "Does it matter that Joan's voices are somewhat unpalatable? It does, of course, if we want Joan's desires and values to match our own. Being able to stomach her inspiration is then of the utmost importance, for if we can't, we will have to season it or cut away the spoiled parts or spit it out. To some extent we all treat Joan this way. She is a hero, and heroes are receptacles for our love or our hatred. But she is also a historical figure with a solidity and a reality all her own" (Smith, 2007, ch. 10).

Her case brings together many of the themes this chapter will follow through other traditions: The way culturally available images and narratives shape what is seen and heard; the power of institutions to validate or pathologise inner experience and the capacity of hallucinatory phenomena to migrate from individual consciousness into collective memory, theology and art. In this sense, Joan's encounter with the hidden king at Chinon is not just a dramatic anecdote, but an emblem of the broader question at stake: When someone claims to see or hear what others cannot, who gets to decide whether this is madness, deception or the voice of the gods?

HEARING THE GODS: THE *ILIAD* AND THE BICAMERAL MIND

Homer's *Iliad* offers a very different landscape from Joan of Arc's France, yet it is just as densely populated with commanding voices and intrusive presences. Again and again, warriors act because a god has spoken to them, appeared before them or seized their thoughts; the poem's world is one in which hearing and seeing the divine is a routine part of decision-making rather than an unusual or pathological event. When Athena grabs Achilles by the hair to stop him from killing Agamemnon, he hears her voice and obeys without any question that this is an external, authoritative agent. When Apollo deceives Hector by taking the form and voice of his ally Deïphobos,

Hector treats the encounter as straightforward social perception: There is no hint that voices or apparitions might be misfirings of his own mind. The *Iliad* thus stages a kind of auditory and visual permeability, in which gods drop into human awareness through words and images that are experienced as real, binding and public—even when, within the story-world, no one else can perceive them.

It was this aspect of the Homeric epics that fascinated Julian Jaynes, a Princeton psychologist who in 1976 published the much-discussed book, *The Origin of Consciousness in the Breakdown of the Bicameral Mind*. Jaynes, who spent much of his career thinking about animal consciousness, introspection and historical psychology, proposed an audacious thesis: That what modern people take for granted as a unified, self-reflective consciousness was not a timeless human constant, but a cultural and neurological achievement that emerged only a few millennia ago. Before this "breakdown", he argued, human cognition was organised in a fundamentally different way, which he called bicameral—literally, "two-chambered". On this view, ancient people did not introspect or narrate their own mental life as "I"; instead, decisions and impulses were experienced as commands heard from outside, often in the guise of gods, ancestors or chiefs. As Jaynes (2000, p. 75) explained, in the bicameral mind, "volition, planning, initiative is organized with no consciousness whatever and then 'told' to the individual in his familiar language, sometimes with the visual aura of a familiar friend or authority figure or 'god', or sometimes as a voice alone. The individual obeyed these hallucinated voices because he could not 'see' what to do by himself".

Jaynes read the *Iliad* as key evidence for his theory of the bicameral mind. He observed how rarely its characters show inner monologue, instead attributing major decisions to divine voices that appear, command and vanish. Rather than treating this as poetic convention, Jaynes proposed it reflected a distinct cognitive style: Under stress or uncertainty, one hemisphere of the brain produced verbal output experienced by the other as an external voice. These "voices of the gods", he argued, once guided behaviour and maintained social order before introspective consciousness emerged. The *Iliad's* world, where deliberation is minimal and divine instruction constant, thus preserves a psychological fossil record of bicameral mentality.

Jaynes placed the breakdown of this mental organisation in the second millennium BCE. As societies grew more complex and unstable through migration and catastrophe, the once-consistent voices of the gods became unreliable. People needed new ways to regulate action and identity, prompting the rise of self-reflective consciousness, law and philosophy. Later texts like the *Odyssey* and Hebrew prophetic writings show a new interiority—characters doubt, hesitate and self-examine—signalling that divine voices were now residual, sometimes troubling phenomena rather than the foundation of mentality.

This narrative naturally resonated with modern psychology's engagement with hallucinations. Jaynes was among the first to suggest that what clinicians call auditory hallucinations may originate in ordinary neurocognitive operations that once served adaptive ends. Modern patients who hear voices might unwittingly experience vestiges of mechanisms that ancient people experienced as divine communication. In that context, hearing a guiding voice would not be pathologised but seen as participation in a shared, animated cosmos. Jaynes reframed voices not as symptoms of disorder but as echoes of an older mode of social and perceptual organisation.

This perspective has quietly supported movements such as the Hearing Voices Network and related qualitative research emphasising that auditory experiences need not signify psychosis. Many voice-hearers describe them as spiritually or personally meaningful, and their impact depends on interpretation and integration rather than content alone. Jaynes's hypothesis offers these movements a kind of "deep historical validation": If hearing voices was once structurally normal, then the modern presumption of pathology is not inevitable. His ideas have therefore attracted clinicians and anthropologists seeking frameworks where voice-hearing represents variation within human cognition rather than categorical abnormality.

Yet the bicameral hypothesis has drawn extensive criticism. Classicists and historians of religion argue that reading the *Iliad* as literal evidence of ancient neurology misinterprets its genre (Riahi, 2014). Epic poetry externalises emotion and motivation by personifying them as gods; divine dialogue dramatises conflict, not necessarily the absence of introspection. Likewise, prophetic voices or visions may function as rhetorical or theological devices, not records of hallucinations. The lack of explicit self-talk in early texts does not prove it was absent in consciousness.

Neuroscientists also challenge Jaynes's claim that the brain reorganised itself radically within a few thousand years (Cavanna et al., 2007). The known evolution of the human nervous system suggests that hemispheric specialisation and language networks long predated recorded history. There is no evidence that humans once lacked introspection or that hemispheric processes functioned as two quasi-independent "chambers". Modern neuropsychology explains auditory hallucinations through mechanisms such as misattributed inner speech, predictive-processing errors and aberrant connectivity—without invoking a vanished mental architecture.

Methodological issues further weaken Jaynes's case. He selected examples that fit his model—scenes of divine command—while minimising passages showing reflection or motive attribution. When he did encounter introspective moments, he treated them as signs of transitional breakdown, a move that renders the theory unfalsifiable. Cross-cultural generalisations pose similar problems: Extrapolating from a few literatures to a global history of consciousness neglects the vast diversity of symbolic traditions.

Despite these flaws, Jaynes's work remains influential because it dramatises how perception and cultural meaning intertwine. In the *Iliad*, hearing a god is not a private symptom but a narrative and social event that reorganises authority and action. Jaynes amplified this insight into a full model of cognition historically structured around auditory guidance. Even if that regime never existed literally, his insistence that mental experience is historically and culturally plastic remains valuable. It challenges reductionist views that treat hallucinations as purely neurological artifacts, untouched by interpretive context.

Clinically, Jaynes's legacy is ambivalent. His specific bicameral model lacks empirical support and cannot explain modern psychosis. Yet the questions he raised—about how consciousness evolves, how societies define "normal" experience and how structured inner dialogue can serve adaptive functions—continue to resonate. By reminding psychology that the boundaries between divine inspiration, moral command and pathological voice are culturally drawn, Jaynes's work keeps open a vital conversation about the historical imagination of the mind.

VOICES, VISIONS AND THE SACRED: RELIGIOUS USES OF HALLUCINATORY EXPERIENCE

Across religious traditions, voices and visions occupy a privileged, but often contested, position as channels through which the sacred addresses human beings. In the three major monotheistic religions, scriptural narratives repeatedly present auditory and visual experiences as decisive moments of revelation, guidance and correction, while later communities argue over how such experiences should be evaluated. In Judaism, for example, the call of Moses at the burning bush is explicitly framed as hearing God speak from within a visual sign that is both ordinary (a shrub) and extraordinary (the fire that does not consume it), and the prophetic literature is saturated with formulae such as "the word of the Lord came to me" (Jeremiah 1:1), which portray speech-like encounters that direct the prophet's message and actions. In Christianity, key moments—Mary's annunciation, Paul's conversion on the road to Damascus, Peter's rooftop vision in Acts—turn on voices, lights and images that break into ordinary perception and reconfigure the believer's understanding of God's purposes. Islam, too, is founded on an auditory experience: Muhammad's reception of the Qur'an through the angel Jibrīl (Gabriel), initially experienced as a terrifying constriction and an overwhelming command to "recite", later interpreted as the archetype of prophetic audition. In all three cases, the religious tradition retrospectively treats these events not as private anomalies, but as world-defining revelations, yet the phenomenological language—hearing a voice, seeing a figure, being addressed by an invisible presence—remains strikingly close to what contemporary psychology would classify, descriptively, as hallucinatory experience.

Greek and Roman religious life makes the link between altered perception and institutional authority even more explicit, particularly in divinatory settings. At Delphi, the Pythia's utterances, produced in a state that ancient authors variously describe as frenzy, possession or inspired speech, were taken as the voice of Apollo himself, mediated through a human body and then interpreted by priests (Wood, 2004). Other oracles at Dodona, Claros and elsewhere combined visual signs—the rustling of oak leaves, the movement of sacred birds, the behaviour of sacrificial entrails—with occasionally reported auditory phenomena, collapsing the distinction between perceiving the environment and perceiving the god. Roman religion integrated these practices into a bureaucratic system of augury and haruspicy, where specialists scrutinised omens and prodigies, sometimes including reports of visionary dreams or apparitions, as part of state decision-making. In such contexts, the question was not whether a voice or vision had occurred in a strictly neurological sense; what mattered was whether the community regarded it as a valid sign from the divine order, and how it should be weighed against other sources of guidance.

In so-called "Oriental" or Asian religious traditions, voices and visions play equally complex roles, although they are often embedded within broader frameworks of meditation, trance and cosmology. Early Buddhist texts record the Buddha being tempted by Māra, a figure who appears in visual and auditory forms, and later Buddhist hagiographies describe monks and mystics encountering bodhisattvas or hearing teachings while in meditative absorption or dreams (Nichols, 2019). In certain strands of Tibetan Buddhism, visionary experiences during advanced practices such as dream yoga or the bardo teachings are actively cultivated and interpreted as encounters with deities or luminous forms that reveal the nature of mind, rather than as perceptual errors needing correction. Hindu traditions preserve a wide range of experiences described as "*darśan*"—literally, seeing a deity or holy person—which can include spontaneous visions of gods, goddesses or gurus that convey reassurance, instruction or blessing (Eck, 1998). Here again, the phenomenological vocabulary overlaps with what clinical language would call hallucinations, yet the cultural framing defines them as moments of heightened reality, not departures from it.

Within monotheistic traditions, such experiences often become focal points of intra-religious dispute. In Judaism, the rabbinic period saw a gradual "closing of prophecy", with later claims to direct divine speech treated with suspicion, precisely because of the need to stabilise doctrine and authority. Christian history is full of debates over mystics who reported visions of Christ, Mary or saints: some, like Teresa of Ávila, were canonised and their experiences defended as authentic; others were condemned as heretical, deluded or demonically deceived.

A specifically demonological reading of unusual experiences runs alongside, and sometimes against, more affirmative religious interpretations. In medieval and early modern Christian Europe, for instance, vivid inner voices or apparitions that deviated from accepted doctrine could be interpreted not as divine but as diabolical—temptations, obsessions or outright possession—especially when they led to disobedience, heresy or social disruption. Canon law, pastoral manuals and witchcraft treatises all contain criteria for discerning spirits, often warning that Satan could mimic angelic appearances or speak in pious language to mislead the faithful. Over time, these demonological frameworks contributed to the stigmatisation of voice-hearing and visionary states, since claiming to "hear something others cannot" could mark a person not only as holy or inspired, but also as morally suspect, spiritually endangered or a potential threat to the community (Sluhovsky, 2007).

This demonological lens also shaped later attitudes that persist into secular modernity. The association between hallucinations and evil spirits left a cultural residue in which hearing voices can still be linked, in popular imagination, to dangerousness, moral weakness or being "possessed", even when the explicit theology has faded. Early psychiatric authors complained that families delayed seeking help because they interpreted symptoms as sorcery, jinn or the devil's work, while some contemporary patients, especially in strongly religious milieus, continue to fear that disclosing voices will lead to accusations of demonic influence rather than offers of support. From a psychological perspective, this history matters because it shows how conceptualising anomalous experience as contact with malign supernatural agents magnifies shame and secrecy, discourages help-seeking and can justify coercive interventions framed as exorcism rather than care.

Likewise, Islamic scholars developed elaborate criteria for distinguishing between true dreams or visions (ru'yā) and satanic or nafs-based illusions, and generally insisted that no new revelation could abrogate the Qur'an, thus curbing the doctrinal authority of later visionaries even when their experiences were respected (Sirriyeh, 2015). In each case, the same kind of experience—hearing a voice, seeing a figure—can be construed as decisive evidence for divine favour, as a harmless personal consolation or as a dangerously misleading hallucination, depending on theological commitments and institutional needs.

Shamanic and possession traditions, both within and outside the major religions, bring another layer. In many Indigenous cultures, shamans report learning their songs, techniques and diagnoses from spirits that appear in altered states induced by fasting, drumming or psychoactive substances. The voices and visions here are explicitly functional: They provide information about the causes of illness, the location of game or the state of the dead, and their reality is judged pragmatically by their efficacy. Possession cults—whether Afro-Brazilian Candomblé, Haitian Vodou or Sufi dhikr practices that include trance—often involve participants hearing divine or spirit voices through their own mouths or those of mediums, blurring the line between internal and external perception. From a psychological standpoint, these are organised, culturally patterned states in which hallucinatory experiences are expected and positively valued; from within the tradition, they are moments when the sacred takes over human agency.

Because voices and visions are so deeply implicated in religious authority, their status is not merely an academic question. If someone claims to have seen an angel or heard God's command, the apologetic or polemical value of that claim depends heavily on whether the experience is framed as a genuine supernatural intervention or as "merely" a hallucination, perhaps arising from stress, illness or suggestion. Religious proponents may appeal to the sincerity, moral fruits or transformative power of the experience as signs of its divine origin, while skeptics may interpret the same features as products of psychological need or social pressure. For psychologists, this terrain is ethically delicate. Retrospectively "diagnosing" historical or scriptural figures—for example, labelling a medieval visionary as schizophrenic or an ecstatic prophet as epileptic—usually outruns the available evidence, since biographical details are sparse, heavily mediated by theological agendas and filtered through centuries of transmission. Any confident claim that religious figures like Isaiah, Paul or Al-Hallāj "had temporal lobe epilepsy" or "suffered from psychosis" or simply "experiences hallucinations" risks projecting modern categories onto very different conceptual worlds.

Nevertheless, psychologists and psychiatrists are sometimes drawn into these debates, not to arbitrate the truth of religious doctrines, but to clarify how certain claims about experience intersect with contemporary knowledge. A recurring example is the argument, advanced by some Christian apologists, that post-resurrection appearances of Jesus could not have been hallucinations because hallucinations are private and there are no collective hallucinations (Wright, 2008). This claim is rhetorically powerful, but scientifically inaccurate. While strictly identical, cinema-like experiences shared in every detail by many people are rare, there is abundant evidence for group-level phenomena in which multiple individuals report related perceptual experiences in a shared context—phenomena often discussed under the headings of mass psychogenic illness, mass suggestion or crowd-induced hallucinations.

In reported Marian apparitions such as Fátima or Medjugorje, for instance, some witnesses describe seeing or hearing the Virgin Mary while others in the same crowd report nothing unusual, and still others experience more ambiguous sensations, such as dancing suns or changes in light. Social psychologists have documented how strong expectations, emotional arousal and suggestive leadership can produce converging reports of anomalous perceptions in groups, even when no corresponding external stimulus can be verified. Historical cases of "dancing manias" in medieval Europe, outbreaks of laughter or shaking in schools and factories and mass UFO sightings that later lacked physical corroboration, all point to the capacity of human groups to co-construct and share unusual experiences that feel real to participants (Bartholomew, 2001). These need not be identical frame-by-frame hallucinations, but they challenge any simple assertion that hallucinations are strictly solitary and therefore cannot underlie religiously significant group experiences.

The upshot for a psychology of hallucinations is not that religious voices and visions can be neatly sorted into categories of "real" and "unreal", but that they exemplify how perception-like experiences without obvious external stimuli are woven into systems of meaning, authority and dispute. Claims about what groups of people can or cannot experience together, whether in ancient Palestine, medieval Europe or modern pilgrimage sites, need to be evaluated in light of what is known about individual and collective perception. At the same time, any attempt to retroactively diagnose or debunk the founding visions of living traditions must reckon with the limits of historical evidence and the ethical implications of pathologising the sacred.

FROM DEMONS TO DIAGNOSIS: THE NINETEENTH-CENTURY MEDICAL TURN

The nineteenth century marks a decisive shift in how voices and visions were understood, moving from primarily theological or moral frameworks towards medical, psychological and neurological ones. Experiences that earlier might have been attributed to demons or divine inspirations were increasingly reframed as objects of scientific description: Symptoms to be classified, localised in the brain and linked to specific disease entities. This "medical turn" did not entirely banish older religious interpretations, but it introduced a new, durable vocabulary in which hallucinations became central to diagnosis and theorising in psychiatry and neurology.

Jean-Étienne Dominique Esquirol—a student of the renowned reformer Philippe Pinel and a key figure in early French psychiatry—is often credited with giving hallucinations their modern conceptual shape (Porter, 1987). Writing in the early nineteenth century, he sought to clarify confusion in clinical language by distinguishing hallucinations from illusions and by locating their source in the mind rather than in the sense organs. Esquirol described illusions as "sensorial errors", distortions of real sensory input influenced by passions or ideas, whereas hallucinations were experiences occurring "without an external object", an involuntary exercise of memory and imagination that nonetheless carried the vividness of perception. This distinction allowed physicians to discuss people who saw or heard things in the absence of stimuli without assuming demonic influence or deliberate deceit, and it supported Esquirol's broader nosology of monomanias—partial insanities in which one domain of mental life was deranged while others remained intact. Crucially, he acknowledged that hallucinations could occur in otherwise "sane" individuals, opening conceptual space for non-psychotic voice-hearing and vision without automatically equating it with total derangement.

A generation later, Alexandre-Jacques-François Brière de Boismont extended this medicalising project through a broad empirical survey of "hallucinations or apparitions", published in the 1840s (Berrios, 1996). Trained as a physician, he collected case histories from hospitals, asylums and everyday life, including religious visions, spectral encounters, bereavement-related apparitions and experiences of voices among both patients and otherwise healthy individuals. What is striking in his work is the attempt to treat apparitions not as curiosities or mere anecdotes but as phenomena that could be systematically gathered, compared and classified, anticipating later epidemiological work on hallucinations in the general population. He emphasised situational and psychological factors—fatigue, grief, fever, sensory deprivation, intense religious emotion—as conditions that favoured hallucinations, pushing further away from strictly demonological accounts. At the same time, he documented many cases in which people experienced transient voices or visions and yet functioned otherwise normally, reinforcing the idea that hallucinations are not synonymous with global insanity. In Brière de Boismont's hands, hallucinations become both clinical signs and human experiences that intersect with mourning, devotion and crisis, rather than mere markers of madness.

By the late nineteenth century, the medical turn in hallucinations had become increasingly entangled with neurology and experimental psychology. Italian psychiatrist Augusto Tamburini, professor at the University of Modena and director of the San Lazzaro Asylum, was a central figure in this development. Engaged in research on cerebral localisation, Tamburini argued that the theory of hallucinations could not achieve real certainty until the sensory centres of the brain—the "ultimate central termination" of sensory pathways—were identified and understood (Scull, 2015). He and colleagues combined clinical observation with experimental methods, including hypnotism and suggestion, to provoke or modulate perceptual anomalies and thereby infer their neural underpinnings. Hypnotic experiments showed that suggestion could induce sensory experiences that subjects reported as real, yet were clearly generated within controlled conditions. These studies reinforced the idea that hallucinations could be produced by perturbations of the nervous system, whether spontaneous or experimentally induced, and thus were proper topics for physiological investigation, while simultaneously highlighting the role of interpersonal influence and expectation in shaping what people perceive.

As the century turned, Eugen Bleuler's work on schizophrenia consolidated many of these earlier threads into a new diagnostic framework. In his 1911 monograph *Dementia Praecox or the Group of Schizophrenias*, Bleuler recast what was then called "dementia praecox" as "schizophrenia", emphasising not inevitable deterioration but a characteristic "splitting" of psychic functions. Hallucinations were not, for Bleuler, the primary defining feature—he reserved that place for his "four As" (disturbances of associations, affect, ambivalence and autism)—yet auditory and other hallucinations were central among the accessory symptoms that gave schizophrenia its clinical profile. Drawing on earlier French and German work, he treated hallucinations as genuine perceptual phenomena, but linked them to affectively charged complexes and disturbances in associative processes. Voices were not random noise; they often expressed conflicts, fears and preoccupations, sometimes in symbolic or fragmentary form. Once schizophrenia was established as a key diagnostic category, hallucinations became widely regarded—especially in the first half of the twentieth century—as hallmarks of severe mental illness, cementing a public association between voice-hearing and madness that continues to shape stigma.

Modern psychology has been largely shaped by the legacy of Sigmund Freud, and although his contributions to this landscape were more oblique, they remained nonetheless influential. Although not primarily a theorist of hallucinations, Freud interpreted them, especially in psychosis, as regressions to more primitive modes of mental functioning, in which internal wishes or fears break through the barrier between fantasy and perception. His analysis approaches persecutory and religious hallucinations as derivatives of repressed libidinal dynamics and defensive operations, rather than as mere products of defective sensory processing (Freud, 2014). Psychoanalytic theory thus added a further layer to the medical turn: Hallucinations could be viewed as meaningful communications from the unconscious, structured like symptoms or dreams, and therefore available to interpretation as well as to neurological explanation. This psychodynamic perspective coexisted uneasily with biologically oriented models, but it deepened the sense that hallucinations are not only events in the brain, but also expressions within a psychological economy of desire, fear, guilt and identity.

The same period also saw hallucinations increasingly treated as research tools. Neurologists and experimental psychologists used them to probe questions about sensory processing, cerebral localisation and the relation between perception and imagination. Hypnosis studies, psychophysical experiments on after-images and sensory thresholds, and early brain lesion research all exploited hallucinations and related phenomena to test hypotheses about the nervous system. Organisations such as the Society for Psychical Research collected reports of apparitions and crisis visions using quasi-scientific methods, reflecting a widespread fascination with "seeing what is not there" across both mainstream medicine and fringe psychical science. Hallucinations thus migrated from the margins of theology and folklore to the centre of scientific inquiry, acting as boundary objects between psychiatry, neurology, psychology and parapsychology.

Ultimately, this medical turn had ambivalent consequences for the social meaning of hallucinations. On the one hand, relocating them from religious approaches to medicine could be humanising: People who heard distressing voices or saw terrifying figures might be treated as patients in need of care rather than as witches, sinners, or frauds. On the other hand, tightly linking hallucinations to severe mental illnesses such as schizophrenia risked pathologising a wide range of unusual experiences and reinforcing associations between voice-hearing and dangerousness.

HALLUCINATIONS AS CULTURAL AND ARTISTIC INSPIRATION

As the focus shifts from religious and medical settings to the wider cultural field, hallucinations continue to function as powerful devices for organising meaning, but now their authority and value are negotiated largely through aesthetic rather than theological or diagnostic frameworks. Literature, in particular, has long treated visions and voices as a way of making interior life visible: Romantic and post-Romantic writers repeatedly linked hallucinatory experience to artistic genius and psychological extremity, with William Blake's reports of conversing with angels and Old Testament prophets blurring the line between mystical encounter and poetic invention, and his illuminated books presenting figures and scenes he explicitly described as "visions". In the nineteenth century, Edgar Allan Poe and Fyodor Dostoevsky used hallucinatory episodes to dramatise guilt, delirium or seizure-related states, anticipating later clinical accounts of alcohol withdrawal and temporal-lobe phenomena, while twentieth-century modernists such as Virginia Woolf and Samuel Beckett rendered intrusive voices and uncanny presences as part of the ordinary fabric of consciousness, sometimes drawing on their own experiences of depression or psychosis, sometimes on emerging psychiatric vocabularies.

Visual art has an equally intricate relationship with hallucinatory experience, ranging from explicit depictions of visions to stylistic experiments that mimic altered perception. Medieval and early modern Christian images of the temptations of Saint Anthony present swarms of grotesque creatures and hybrid forms that can be read, in retrospect, as visualisations of nightmare and delirium, even though contemporaries understood them primarily as spiritual assaults. In the nineteenth century, artists such as Francisco Goya and later Vincent van Gogh produced works that have been retrospectively linked to hallucinations associated with illness, intoxication, or affective disturbance—Goya's late "Black Paintings" and van Gogh's swirling skies and distorted perspectives have invited speculation about visual aura, psychosis or substance use, even if definitive diagnosis remains elusive. The twentieth-century Surrealists, including Salvador Dalí and Max Ernst, deliberately courted hallucination-like imagery through techniques such as the "paranoiac-critical" method and automatism, seeking to short-circuit rational control and give pictorial form to dreamlike or intrusive mental content.

Music and film bring their own modalities to the representation of hallucinations. In opera and art song, mad scenes—from Donizetti's Lucia di Lammermoor to Schoenberg's Erwartung—use fragmented melodies, abrupt shifts and orchestral colour to suggest a mind overwhelmed by voices or visions, reinforcing the Romantic stereotype of madness as tragic excess. Popular music has long mined psychedelic and psychotic imagery, whether in explicitly drug-linked work like The Beatles' *Lucy in the Sky with Diamonds* and Jimi Hendrix's *Purple Haze*, or in later genres where hearing voices becomes a metaphor for alienation and creativity alike. Cinema, with its control over image and sound, has developed highly stylised ways of depicting hallucinations—from the subjective camera and sound design in films such as *A Beautiful Mind* and *Black Swan*, which place viewers inside the protagonist's altered perception, to horror and fantasy films that blur the boundary between diegetic reality and hallucinatory sequences. These audiovisual strategies can either pathologise hallucinations, presenting them as terrifying harbingers of breakdown or romanticise them as gateways to hidden truths, depending on genre conventions and directorial choices.

Hallucinations, then, do not float free of history, culture or meaning, but they are also not reducible to them. The same kinds of experiences that have been hailed as revelation, feared as witchcraft or medicalised as symptoms all depend, at some level, on how the brain constructs a world from partial and ambiguous signals. It is time, then, to move from this wide historical and cultural canvas to the underlying machinery that makes such experiences possible: In the next chapter, we will turn from saints, spirits and social judgements to the brain itself, tracing how predictive processing, sensory pathways and neuromodulatory systems can generate experiences of seeing and hearing what is not there, and how these same processes sometimes overshoot their mark in ways that feel so convincingly real.

2

HALLUCINATIONS
AND THE BRAIN

In 1760, the Swiss naturalist Charles Bonnet published *Analytical essay on the faculties of the soul*, in which he described an unsettling change in his 87-year-old grandfather, Charles Lullin, a retired magistrate in Geneva. After cataract operations had left Lullin almost completely blind, he began to report seeing men and women in elaborate dress, birds perched on furniture, carriages rolling past, buildings, tapestries and intricate scaffolding patterns, all in perfect clarity and with no corresponding objects in the room. Bonnet emphasised that his grandfather was otherwise in good health, with intact judgement and memory, and that he recognised these visions as unreal even as they appeared with the force of genuine perception. Years later, Bonnet himself would experience similar "phantom visions" as his own eyesight deteriorated, reinforcing his conviction that such hallucinations could arise in lucid, psychologically intact people whose sensory input had been severely compromised (Draaisma, 2009).

Bonnet's careful documentation of these episodes, which would only much later be gathered under the label "Charles Bonnet syndrome", posed a quiet but radical challenge to prevailing assumptions about hallucinations. His observations

DOI: 10.4324/9781003784890-3

suggested that the brain does not merely receive the world but can generate richly structured, perception-like experiences on its own, especially when normal sensory signals fall silent or become patchy.

Accounts like these unsettle intuitive models of vision and hearing. Yet the experiences of visually impaired but otherwise healthy people with vivid complex hallucinations point in a different direction. They suggest that the brain is constantly generating predictions, templates and patterns, and that these internally generated images can flood consciousness when incoming data are weak or ambiguous. In such cases, hallucinations are not arbitrary intrusions but the visible traces of an active system that would rather over-interpret than leave a gap.

The same logic appears, in a more troubling form, in conditions far removed from gentle retirement. A young man with schizophrenia hears a running commentary on his actions in what sounds like a familiar voice, yet neurological examination and hearing tests show nothing wrong with his ears. A woman emerging from a period of extreme sleep deprivation begins to see shadowy figures in her peripheral vision, always vanishing when she turns her head. A patient with Parkinson's disease reports small animals scurrying across the floor, knowing they are not real but feeling as though her visual world has become porous and unreliable. Each of these situations forces clinicians and researchers to ask the same question: What is the brain doing such that its own productions are experienced as if they came from outside?

This chapter turns from the historical and cultural canvases of the previous one to the biological and cognitive processes that make hallucinations possible. The focus now shifts to the neural and psychological mechanisms that generate them. The aim is not to reduce rich subjective experiences to crude "brain glitches", but to understand how normal perception is constructed, where it can go awry and why certain patterns of breakdown repeat across many diverse conditions.

BUILDING PERCEPTUAL REALITY: NEUROBIOLOGY OF HALLUCINATIONS

Perception begins as a physical event: light strikes the retina, sound waves vibrate the eardrum, chemicals bind to receptors in the nose or tongue, pressure deforms the skin. But the flow from outside world to inner experience is never simply a one-way relay of facts (Sprevak & Smith, 2023). The brain is not a camera that records; it is a storyteller that constructs. Signals are interpreted, compared with past experience and fitted into an ongoing narrative about what is happening "out there". When hallucinations occur, they do not arise from an alien system bolted onto perception; they emerge from the very machinery that usually allows a person to navigate the world with confidence. The same networks that ordinarily support seeing, hearing and feeling can, under certain conditions, generate perception-like experiences without appropriate input. In this sense, hallucinations are less an add-on to perception than an amplification of its constructive tendencies.

As neuroscientist Anil Seth (2021) has influentially argued, normal perception can be understood as a form of "controlled hallucination", in which the brain actively generates top-down predictions about the causes of sensory input and then keeps these in check by continually comparing them with incoming signals. From this perspective, clinical hallucinations arise when these internally generated models are insufficiently constrained by sensory evidence, so that the same constructive processes that usually yield a stable, shared world instead produce experiences that drift away from the current environment while still feeling fully real.

Perception begins in the brain's primary sensory cortices, where incoming information from the senses first arrives. The primary visual cortex in the occipital lobes processes signals from the eyes, the primary auditory cortex along the upper temporal lobe handles sounds and the somatosensory cortex in the parietal lobes interprets touch and body sensations. These inputs travel through the thalamus—an egg-shaped structure deep in the brain that serves as a central relay station—before reaching their respective cortical areas. From there, the information moves on to secondary and association cortices, where simple sensory features such as edges and movement in vision or pitch and timing in hearing are integrated into coherent images, words and experiences. Brain imaging studies show that during hallucinations, these same sensory regions become active, even though no external stimulus is present (Zmigrod et al., 2016). For example, visual hallucinations often activate visual association areas, while auditory hallucinations engage auditory and language regions. In essence, hallucinations trigger the brain's sensory maps in much the same way real perceptions do, even when the eyes or ears are silent (Abid et al., 2016).

This overlap is particularly striking in auditory verbal hallucinations, the experience of hearing voices. Functional imaging studies of people who hear voices during psychosis, as well as non-clinical voice-hearers, consistently show that language-related regions—such as parts of the superior temporal gyrus (involved in speech perception) and inferior frontal gyrus or Broca's area (involved in speech production)—become active when a voice is reported, even in the absence of external sound (Wible et al., 2009). Some work finds similar engagement of temporo-parietal regions associated with Wernicke's area, which supports comprehension of spoken language (Hoffman & Hampson, 2012). These observations help explain why voices often have recognizable accents, gender and emotional tone, and why they can sound as clear as someone speaking nearby. The networks that normally allow a person to listen and talk are, in effect, talking to themselves. The experience feels imposed because the brain systems that tag an event as "self-generated" versus "coming from outside" are not correctly marking the source.

Beyond these cortical territories, deeper structures help decide which signals reach awareness and how much weight they carry. The thalamus, sitting near the centre of the brain, routes sensory information to appropriate cortical areas and plays a key role in filtering and prioritising input. Experimental and clinical work suggests that when thalamocortical circuits become dysregulated—through neurodegenerative change, substances or psychotic processes—sensory gating may be altered in ways that favour internally generated activity over external signals (Onofrj et al., 2023).

The limbic system, which includes structures such as the hippocampus and amygdala, contributes another dimension by attaching emotional weight and autobiographical context to what is perceived. Meta-analyses of hallucinations across different studies show involvement not only of sensory cortices but also of hippocampal, paralimbic and prefrontal regions (Rollins et al., 2019). This helps explain why hallucinations are rarely neutral flickers of sensation. Voices may arrive with a crushing sense of condemnation or reassurance; a visual figure may feel menacing, familiar or sacred. The amygdala and related regions help tag stimuli—real or hallucinatory—with threat, salience or reward value (Ford et al., 2015), while the hippocampus contributes elements of memory (Amad et al., 2014), leading to content that echoes past relationships, traumas or cultural imagery. From the person's perspective, the emotional force of the experience is part of what makes it real; the brain systems that normally flag events as important are signalling that this perception matters.

Another important player is the striatum, a cluster of deep brain structures that sit beneath the cortex and form part of the basal ganglia (Cassidy et al., 2018). It is richly supplied with dopamine-releasing neurons, making it a key hub for this chemical messenger. Brain-imaging studies in psychosis repeatedly show that when dopamine activity in mesolimbic and striatal circuits is elevated, hallucinations and delusions become more likely (McCutcheon et al., 2018). A helpful way to think about dopamine in this context is as a "teaching" or "highlighting" signal. It helps the brain decide which patterns in the world to pay attention to and which events are worth learning from. When dopamine surges, the brain effectively marks a stimulus or an internal event as important, something to be tracked and remembered.

Recent animal work has pushed this idea further by generating controlled, hallucination-like experiences in laboratory settings.

In experiments where a very faint tone might or might not be played, researchers increased dopamine levels in the striatum, either using drugs such as ketamine or by directly stimulating dopamine-releasing cells. Under these conditions, mice started to respond as if they had heard the tone even when no sound was presented at all (Lakshminarasimhan et al., 2025). Computational models of these tasks suggest what is going on behind the scenes (Sterzer et al., 2018). When dopamine is abnormally high, the brain leans more heavily on its own expectations and not enough on the actual sensory evidence arriving from the outside world. Perception becomes biased towards what the system predicts should be there, rather than what is truly present. From this vantage point, hallucinations can be understood as the lived outcome of a brain that is over-learning from its own predictions, allowing anticipated patterns to override reality.

The way these brain regions are wired together also matters for how hallucinations arise. Bundles of nerve fibres known as white-matter tracts, such as the arcuate fasciculus that links frontal and temporal language areas, and longer-range connections between sensory, frontal and cingulate regions, determine how easily activity in one area can influence another.

Imaging studies that track the structure of these pathways suggest that people who often hear voices can, in some cases, have stronger connections between regions involved in producing and perceiving speech than people who do not report such experiences. Brain scans taken while hallucinations are actually occurring show that several key areas tend to fire together: Parts of the inferior frontal cortex, auditory cortex, the ventral striatum and the cingulate cortex (Ćurčić-Blake et al., 2017). The more tightly this activity is coupled, the more real and compelling the voices tend to feel. Thinking at this network level shifts the focus from single "hotspots" to patterns of communication across the brain. Hallucinations can be seen as what happens when loops linking expectation, sensation and evaluation start to resonate in particular ways, so that internally driven activity is passed around and amplified until it is experienced as coming from outside.

All of this detail raises a larger question: How does the brain ordinarily construct a stable world from noisy signals, and what changes when hallucinations occur? One influential view treats perception as an ongoing form of inference or hypothesis-testing (Gregory, 1980). On this view, the brain constantly generates predictions about what it is likely to encounter—based on past experience, context and internal needs—and compares these predictions with sensory input. Imagine someone who has lost much of their sight but begins to see vivid scenes and figures. Their eyes now send only fragments of information, yet the visual cortex and surrounding association areas remain active and continue doing what they are built to do—search for patterns and meaning. When normal visual input fades, these brain regions may begin to "free-run", drawing on well-stored templates of faces, rooms, landscapes and other familiar images. At the same time, shifts in thalamocortical communication and in the brain's chemical balance can amplify this internally generated activity until it becomes strong enough to reach conscious awareness. The result is not random visual noise but organised, recognizable images that reveal the visual system's deep inclination towards patterns, people and places.

Something similar can happen in the auditory and emotional systems: A person under intense stress who begins to hear a harsh, critical voice may be experiencing a convergence of overactive language networks, limbic regions that are primed for threat and dopamine-driven biases towards expecting danger or criticism, so that fleeting fragments of inner speech or ambiguous background sounds are more likely to be misread as coming from outside and take the form of an external, hostile commentary rather than being recognised as their own thoughts.

Hallucinations can also emerge in post-traumatic stress disorder (PTSD), where intrusive memories, flashbacks and hypervigilance blur the line between past and present so completely that trauma-related images, sounds or voices are experienced as if they are happening right now rather than being recognised as memories (Lyndon & Corlett, 2020). In some combat veterans, for example, the sound of a car backfiring may not only trigger a flashback but also lead to hearing the echo of gunfire or shouted commands that are not actually present, creating an experience that is phenomenologically close to an auditory hallucination. Similar reports have appeared in survivors of accidents or assaults who see the perpetrator's face in the room or feel their touch on the skin despite knowing, at another level, that they are currently safe.

These mechanisms help to explain an apparent paradox. On the one hand, hallucinations can be deeply idiosyncratic, filled with personal symbolism and autobiographical echoes. On the other hand, across individuals and conditions, certain regularities appear: Voices that comment or command; figures at the edge of vision; animals or strangers in the room; patterns and faces emerging from darkness. The brain is shaped by evolutionary pressures and developmental history to prioritise particular kinds of information—voices, faces, agents and especially potential threats—and its predictive machinery is tuned to detect danger quickly enough to escape predators or other hazards, even at the cost of occasional false alarms. In ancestral environments, a system that over-reacted to rustling in the bushes or a shadow in the periphery could be life-saving, but in modern settings—quiet bedrooms, city streets, hospital wards—the same hypervigilant circuits can misfire or become chronically over-engaged, generating perceptions of threat where none exists. When perception decouples from the environment, it does not wander aimlessly; it tends to generate versions of the stimuli that matter most. The networks that ordinarily support social perception, language and threat detection are therefore the ones most likely to seed hallucinations, because they are the systems the brain most heavily rehearses, expects to use and evolutionarily "prefers" to err on the side of activating.

MECHANISMS OF MISPERCEPTION: MAJOR THEORIES OF HALLUCINATIONS

When people report hallucinations, researchers rarely assume a single cause. Instead, they draw on several overlapping theories that try to show how normal processes of perception, thinking and memory can tip into misperception. Although these accounts highlight different mechanisms—sensory loss, inner speech, memory or prediction—they share a common theme already suggested by authors such as Richard Bentall (1990): Hallucinations are not alien additions to the mind, but exaggerations or distortions of how perception usually works. They are "extreme versions" of everyday constructive perception, pushed beyond the point where reality can easily pull them back.

One of the oldest strands of thinking focuses on what happens when sensory input is reduced or lost. Sensory deafferentation or "release" models, associated with early neurological observations by Charles Bonnet and later developed by authors like Dominic Ffytche (2008) and Alan Zeman (2002), emphasise that sensory regions of the brain can become overactive when normal input is weakened. Deafferentation simply means that the usual incoming signals from the eyes or ears are cut down or cut off. As in the opening story of this chapter, classic descriptions of Charles Bonnet–type experiences involve people with serious eye disease or profound visual loss who begin to see vivid faces, landscapes or small figures that appear and disappear without warning, even though they remain fully lucid and aware that these images are not real. In this framework, visual cortex is no longer tightly driven by retinal input and begins to "release" its own stored patterns—familiar templates for objects and scenes that now bubble up into awareness. A television analogy is helpful: When the signal weakens, the screen does not just go blank; instead, noise and improvised patterns appear. Hallucinations, in this context, are internally generated activity that is normally held in check by continuous sensory input.

When sensory models focus on what happens when input is missing, inner speech and self-monitoring accounts ask what the brain is doing when hearing is perfectly normal. These theories, associated with Chris Frith (1996), Paul Fletcher (2017) and others, suggest that many auditory verbal hallucinations arise when the system that usually keeps track of one's own inner speech stops working properly. Most adults spend a surprising amount of time talking silently to themselves, using an inner voice to plan the day, rehearse conversations or comment on what they are doing. This inner voice is built using the brain's ordinary language machinery: Regions in the left temporal lobe that process speech and areas in the frontal lobe, such as the inferior frontal gyrus (often called Broca's area), that help put words together. Frith's self-monitoring model proposes that whenever a person prepares to speak—either aloud or in their head—the brain sends a kind of advance warning to auditory regions, telling them that the upcoming "sound" will be self-generated. If this warning signal (sometimes called a corollary discharge) is too weak or mistimed, the inner speech still occurs but is no longer tagged as "mine", so it can be experienced as if it were coming from someone else. On this view, the voices heard in psychosis are produced by the person's own language circuits, but because the monitoring system has failed, they are misattributed to external agents—gods, demons, neighbours, authorities—rather than recognised as self-generated thoughts.

Another set of ideas, associated with Elizabeth Loftus (1993) and Marcia Johnson (1997), and Richard Bentall (1990), takes the same basic logic and asks a broader question: How does the mind keep track of where experiences come from? Source-monitoring and memory-intrusion theories suggest that hallucinations can appear when the internal "labelling system" that marks events as real, imagined, remembered or dreamed starts to fail. Johnson's source-monitoring framework was first developed to explain why people sometimes confuse memories of actual events with things they only pictured or were told about, but Bentall and others have applied it to hallucinations, showing that people who are prone to them are more likely to treat their own thoughts, images or self-generated words as if they came from outside—especially when those inner events are vivid or emotionally charged.

Clinical work on trauma adds that intrusive, sensory-rich memories can erupt into awareness as flashbacks that feel as if they are happening right now, rather than as something safely in the past, blurring the line between remembering and perceiving (Van Der Kolk, 1998). Furthermore, dissociation can disrupt the sense of a continuous, coherent self and a stable context, making it easier for images, feelings or pieces of experience to be felt as if they are happening "to" the person from outside rather than arising within. From this angle, hallucinations look like misfiled experiences: products of memory, imagination or emotion that have been stamped, incorrectly, with the label "here-and-now perception".

Predictive processing and so-called "Bayesian models" offer a simpler way of claiming that the brain is always guessing and then checking. These accounts, developed by authors like Karl Friston (2005), Jakob Hohwy (2025) and Rick Adams (2018), describe the brain as a prediction machine that constantly anticipates what it will see or hear next and compares these guesses with what actually arrives through the senses. When reality does not match the prediction, the difference creates a "prediction error" signal that tells the system something needs to be revised. A key idea is that the brain also decides how much trust, or "precision", to place on its expectations versus on the incoming data. If it trusts its expectations too much, or treats the error signals from the senses as weak or unimportant, then what it expects can override what is actually there. In that situation, a strong expectation of hearing a voice can be enough to make the auditory parts of the brain behave as if a voice were present, even when the ears are getting only faint or unclear sounds. This suggests that prediction and error signals can sometimes get caught in self-reinforcing loops, echoing back and forth in the cortex and giving rise to perceptions that carry on even when the outside evidence clearly says they should stop.

What stands out across these frameworks is how much they have in common despite their different starting points. All treat hallucinations as emerging from ordinary ingredients of mental life—perception, inner speech, memory, imagery, attention and prediction—that are pushed, by circumstance or vulnerability, into extreme territory. On this view, hallucinations are not simply errors to be brushed aside, but revealing experiments of nature: They show what the mind's constructive machinery is capable of when its habits of interpretation and expectation run ahead of the world's ability to constrain them.

A WORKING TAXONOMY OF HALLUCINATIONS

One way to move from theory to practice is to classify hallucinations not only by where they occur in the body or which diagnosis they accompany, but by the mechanisms that seem to drive them. This kind of classification cuts across traditional categories and helps explain why very different people, in very different situations, can report surprisingly similar experiences. It also sits alongside more familiar ways of sorting hallucinations by sensory modality— vision, hearing, touch, smell, taste and bodily sensations—because different mechanisms tend to recruit different senses.

A first grouping centres on sensory-deprivation and release phenomena. Here, the key feature is that the relevant sense organs are providing less input than usual, or that normal sensory signals are intermittently disrupted. In people with profound visual loss, for example, the eyes may transmit only faint, fragmentary information, but visual cortex and higher visual areas remain active and highly organised. In this situation, the visual system is thought to "free-run", drawing on deeply learned patterns—faces, rooms, landscapes, geometric designs—to fill in the gaps, producing detailed visual scenes that have no counterpart in the outside world. Similar release effects can occur in other modalities: Prolonged silence or sudden hearing loss may allow spontaneous activity in auditory cortex to be experienced as music, voices or simple tones; long periods of isolation or sensory monotony can generate a mix of fleeting visual, auditory and tactile impressions as the brain attempts to maintain a continuous stream of experience. Hallucinations in this cluster are organised by the state of the sensory channels: Where the world has fallen quiet, the system generates its own content.

A second grouping draws on hypervigilance, threat-detection and trauma-related mechanisms. The human nervous system is tuned to pick up on potential danger—an angry voice, a looming figure, a sudden touch—and under conditions of chronic threat, this tuning can become exaggerated. People who have lived through prolonged fear or abuse may develop a cortex and limbic system that are primed to expect attack, to over-interpret ambiguous cues as hostile, and to narrow attention onto signs of danger. In such states, ordinary background noise may be heard as footsteps, someone calling one's name, or whispering at the edge of hearing, as the auditory system and threat-detection circuits collaborate to "fill in" a feared scenario. Visual perception can likewise become haunted by expectations of harm: Shadows at the periphery may resolve themselves into figures; fleeting movements can be seen as someone lurking or following, even when no one is there.

A third cluster centres on language and agency-monitoring failures, especially for voices and other auditory verbal phenomena. Here, the person's basic hearing is intact, but the brain systems that produce and track inner speech and self-generated actions become unreliable. The language network—including regions in the left temporal lobe that process speech sounds and frontal areas that help assemble and articulate words—continues to generate streams of inner commentary, questions and responses as it does in everyone. The difference is that the monitoring mechanisms that usually tag this material as "mine" no longer work smoothly. Thoughts can be heard as if they were spoken aloud; inner dialogue can split into multiple "voices" with distinct tones, genders or attitudes; familiar sentences can arrive with the feel of an external broadcast rather than an inner reflection.

In some dissociative states, this fragmentation extends beyond speech: Movements, urges or emotionally laden images may be experienced as imposed by an external agent, producing a sense of being controlled or occupied. Although auditory verbal hallucinations are the most obvious outcome, related failures of agency-monitoring can involve other senses—such as feeling a hand on one's shoulder when the muscle activity and posture are generated from within, or "seeing" one's own mental images as if they were projected into the room. Mechanistically, what ties these experiences together is not the modality but the difficulty in recognising self-generated activity as self-generated.

A fourth group concerns pharmacological and neuromodulatory perturbations—situations where chemicals, whether drugs or disease-related changes, alter how strongly different signals are amplified or dampened in the brain. Psychedelic substances, stimulants, anticholinergic drugs and many prescribed medications can all shift the balance between internal predictions and sensory evidence. In these cases, the classification by mechanism emphasises what has been done to neuromodulatory systems; the sensory profile—visual, auditory, tactile, olfactory—depends on which circuits are most destabilised for that individual.

Alongside these mechanism-based families, it remains useful to consider the sensory modalities involved, because some mechanisms favour particular channels more than others. Visual hallucinations often reflect disturbances in the visual system, whether from sensory loss, drug effects or disease processes that affect how visual cortex predicts and organises input. Auditory hallucinations include not only voices and music but also knocks, bangs, buzzing and more abstract sounds; these tend to track mechanisms involving inner speech, hypervigilance to threat and changes in how salience and prediction are handled in auditory pathways. Tactile or somatic hallucinations—sensations of being touched, insects crawling on the skin, electrical currents, internal movement—feature prominently in some drug-related states, certain neurological conditions and trauma-linked reactions where the body's memory of harm is easily re-evoked.

Olfactory hallucinations illustrate this point especially clearly: Although less common than visual or auditory phenomena, brief, intrusive smells of smoke, gas or cheap perfume can signal focal temporal lobe disturbance rather than a primary psychiatric disorder, and persistent foul or distorted smells may follow damage to the olfactory pathways. In Oliver Sacks' (2013, ch. 8) account of temporal lobe epilepsy in his well-known book *Hallucinations*, one patient described how "there is a disgusting sweet, penetrating odour like very cheap perfume… I am all alone with the smell", an experience that recurs in stereotyped fashion as part of her seizure aura. Such vignettes underscore how, in some conditions, olfactory hallucinations function as highly specific markers of underlying neurological pathology, even when patients or clinicians initially interpret them as environmental threats or signs of mental illness.

Nevertheless, it is important to point out that no single theory of hallucinations can do justice to the sheer variety of what people report. Inner speech models fit many persecutory voices but say little about the smell of smoke in temporal lobe epilepsy; sensory-release accounts illuminate complex visions after visual loss but do not explain second-person commands that echo a person's own critical thoughts. The same applies to classification systems. Sorting hallucinations by sensory modality, by diagnosis or by underlying brain condition each captures something important, yet each leaves out patterns that cut across those boundaries. There will always be experiences that sit awkwardly between categories, or that seem to fit several at once.

What mechanism-based thinking offers is not a final map, but a better starting point for clinical and phenomenological work. When a clinician asks not only "What do you see or hear?" but also "Under what conditions did this start? What else was happening in your body, your life, your environment?", they are already reasoning in mechanism-oriented terms. For researchers and clinicians, this way of thinking does not replace attention to diagnosis, culture or subjective meaning, but it sharpens them. It encourages a habit of asking what has happened to the systems that usually keep perception anchored, and how those specific shifts might be modified, compensated for or integrated, rather than treating all hallucinations as interchangeable symptoms that demand the same response.

Across these models, there is still no full agreement on what hallucinations "really are". Different traditions place inner speech, memory intrusions, predictive failures, sensory release or neuro-modulatory shifts at the centre, and each risks overstating its preferred mechanism. What is increasingly clear, though, is that several mechanisms can operate at once, even within a single person or episode: A trauma-sensitised threat system can colour the content of voices generated by inner-speech circuits, while sensory changes and medication quietly alter the balance between prediction and evidence in the background. The same hallucination may therefore be simultaneously a release phenomenon, a misattributed inner dialogue and a memory-suffused construction. The next chapter turns from this mechanistic landscape to the clinical terrain of psychosis, where these layered processes are woven into patterns of delusion, disorganisation and help-seeking, and where hallucinations become one thread in a much larger diagnostic fabric.

3

HALLUCINATIONS AND PSYCHOSIS

In 1903, a book was published that would come to occupy a central place in the modern understanding of mental illness: *Memoirs of My Nervous Illness*, by German author Daniel Paul Schreber. Written after prolonged hospitalisations in psychiatric institutions, the memoir offers an intricate first-person account of a world reshaped by voices, divine rays and radical bodily transformations. In the decades that followed, these pages—dense with hallucinated speech, visionary experiences and bizarre somatic sensations—became a kind of Rosetta stone for psychiatry and psychoanalysis, a document in which hallucinations and delusions appeared not as scattered curiosities, but as the organising principles of an entire inner universe.

Schreber had been a respected jurist, known for his meticulous reasoning and public composure. In mid-life, however, his world began to split. He reported hearing "voices" that spoke in strange, fragmented German, commenting on his thoughts, mocking his movements and issuing cryptic divine messages. He became convinced that rays emanating from God were penetrating his body, altering his nerves and gradually turning him into a woman destined to repopulate a renewed world. These were not fleeting impressions.

DOI: 10.4324/9781003784890-4

They formed a continuous environment in which he lived for years: Voices that kept up a running commentary, visual and bodily sensations that confirmed his persecution and his chosenness and a thick web of meanings that bound every event to a supernatural plot. As he explained, "all these souls spoke to me as voices more or less at the same time without one knowing of the presence of the others. Everyone who realises that all this is not just the morbid offspring of my fantasy, will be able to appreciate the unholy turmoil they caused in my head" (Schreber & Dinnage, 2000). From the outside, clinicians described a textbook case of paranoid psychosis. From the inside, as his memoir shows, Schreber experienced a coherent—if terrifying and often ecstatic—reality that demanded interpretation rather than simple dismissal.

What makes Schreber's case so enduring is not only its extravagance, but its almost clinical clarity in showing how hallucinations and delusions interlock. The voices he heard did not float in isolation; they belonged to specific agents—God, "nerves of other people", hostile forces—whose intentions he tried to decipher. The bodily changes he felt, from sensations in his genitals to the conviction that his internal organs were being rearranged, anchored a delusional narrative of transformation that explained why the voices had chosen him. In this way, hallucinations become both evidence and fuel: Each new phrase heard, each strange tactile impression, confirmed the broader belief system, while the belief system in turn shaped what was heard and felt.

The afterlife of Schreber's memoir further illustrates how psychotic hallucinations are never purely private events. Sigmund Freud (2014) seized upon the text as a window into psychotic experience, treating Schreber's voices and visions as meaningful derivatives of unconscious conflict and sexual fantasy rather than as meaningless noise. Later psychiatrists read the same pages through different lenses: As classic phenomenology of schizophrenia, as evidence of specific cognitive and perceptual disruptions or as a paradigmatic example of how reality testing can fracture while other intellectual capacities remain intact.

At the centre of Schreber's story lies a question that drives this chapter: What does it mean to say that someone has "lost contact with reality" when their experiences are, in their own terms, so intensely real? In everyday language, psychosis is often reduced to a stereotype of "seeing things" or "hearing voices". Yet Schreber's memoir shows that hallucinations in psychosis are rarely isolated sparks. They entwine with beliefs, moods and social relationships, structuring how a person understands themselves and others. The voices may criticise, command or console; they may speak in tones of persecution or divine mission; they may be resisted, negotiated or obeyed. The task is not only to catalogue these experiences, but to place them within the broader patterns that clinicians call psychosis: Delusions, disorganisation and disturbances of self-experience that together reshape the boundary between inner and outer worlds.

DEFINING PSYCHOSIS AND PLACING HALLUCINATIONS WITHIN IT

Psychosis, in contemporary clinical use, refers less to a single disease and more to a pattern of experiences in which reality testing is compromised (Calabrese & Khalili, 2023). At its core are phenomena such as hallucinations, delusions and marked disorganisation of thought or behaviour, which together signal that a person's usual grip on shared reality has loosened. Rather than standing alone, hallucinations are one thread in this broader disturbance, and their meaning, risk and diagnostic weight depend heavily on the company they keep in a person's mental life.

In modern psychiatry, psychosis is usually defined not by one symptom but by a cluster of characteristic disturbances. Apart from hallucinations, delusions are also likely to be found. Whereas hallucinations involve perceptual experiences, delusions entail fixed, false beliefs that persist despite clear contradictory evidence. In psychosis, disorganised thinking and speech, evident in derailment, incoherence or tangentiality that makes a person's communication difficult to follow, are also central, as are grossly disorganised or catatonic behaviours that appear bizarre, unpredictable or markedly reduced in responsiveness or movement (Bentall & Beck, 2004). Clinicians often encapsulate this picture by saying that psychosis reflects a "loss of contact with reality" (Stephensen, 2025), but this phrase should not be read too literally; people can move in and out of psychotic states, and the "loss" is rarely complete or uniform across all areas of life.

Famous clinical narratives help to ground these abstractions. Consider, for example, John Nash, the mathematician whose life inspired the film *A Beautiful Mind*. Biographical reconstructions highlight how persecutory and grandiose delusions, along with intermittent hallucinations, gradually reorganised his experience: Shadowy conspirators, imagined government plots and voices or presences that seemed to provide privileged information (Nasar, 2011). The hallucinations, where present, did not simply sit beside his beliefs; they provided concrete "evidence" that made an otherwise implausible worldview feel compelling and internally coherent. In this sense, Nash's experience illustrates a common clinical pattern: Psychosis emerges not from hallucinations or delusions in isolation, but from the way perception-like phenomena and fixed beliefs interlock to sustain an alternative reality.

Hallucinations fit naturally within this broader picture because they supply vivid, emotionally charged "data" for altered beliefs. Hearing a voice that issues insults or commands, seeing a threatening figure in an empty room or feeling one's body being manipulated from outside provides exactly the sort of immediate, sensory experience the mind is designed to treat as real. When these experiences arise against a background of suspiciousness, mood disturbance or cognitive fragmentation, they are rapidly woven into delusional explanations: The voice belongs to the secret police, the figure is a demon, the bodily sensations confirm that one has been implanted with a device. Psychosis, in this sense, is not simply hallucinations plus delusions, but a dynamic system in which perception-like events and fixed beliefs continuously shape and reinforce one another.

At the same time, psychosis can occur without prominent hallucinations—for example, in some delusional disorders where belief is the primary disturbance and perception remains largely intact (Munro, 2006). Conversely, as we have already emphasised, hallucinations can occur without psychosis, as in certain neurological syndromes, bereavement-related visions, sleep-related experiences or non-clinical voice-hearing. The term "psychosis" therefore marks a particular configuration: Hallucinations and/or delusions embedded in a more global shift in how reality is appraised, communicated and acted upon, often with marked distress or impairment.

The DSM-5, the main diagnostic manual used by psychiatrists to classify mental disorders, set out how schizophrenia and related psychotic disorders are defined (Association, 2022). They do this by listing key "Criterion A" symptoms for schizophrenia: (1) delusions, (2) hallucinations, (3) disorganised speech, (4) grossly disorganised or catatonic behaviour and (5) negative symptoms such as reduced emotional expression or motivation.

These are often divided into positive and negative symptoms. Positive symptoms are additions to ordinary experience—things "added" to the person's psychological life, such as hallucinations, delusions and disorganised speech or behaviour. Negative symptoms, by contrast, are losses or reductions, including blunted affect, reduced speech, lack of motivation and social withdrawal (Harvey & Walker, 2013). Hallucinations are therefore a classic example of a positive symptom: They bring vivid, perception-like experiences that were not there before, and so play a central role in how psychosis is recognised. To meet diagnostic criteria for schizophrenia, a person must show at least two Criterion A symptoms for a significant part of one month and at least one of them must be a positive symptom. Hallucinations thus occupy a privileged position among the defining features of psychosis, but they are not enough on their own; without additional symptoms (including, often, negative symptoms) and clear evidence of decline in functioning, a diagnosis of schizophrenia cannot be made.

This logic extends across related diagnoses such as schizophreniform disorder, brief psychotic disorder and schizoaffective disorder. Schizophreniform disorder applies when the same symptom pattern is present but the overall duration of disturbance is between one and six months rather than six months or more (Strakowski, 1994), while brief psychotic disorder describes sudden onset of at least one core psychotic symptom, lasting at least one day but less than one month, with eventual full return to premorbid functioning (Fusar-Poli et al., 2022). In all of these, hallucinations can be prominent, yet they must appear in tandem with other psychotic features and a characteristic time course to satisfy DSM-5 criteria. This is precisely why, in many of the better-known case histories—from Nash to Schreber—the diagnostic discussion hinges not only on hallucinatory content, but also on duration, functional impact and the presence of delusions or disorganisation.

Schizoaffective disorder shows how DSM-5 positions hallucinations at the intersection of psychosis and mood. The manual requires an uninterrupted illness during which there is a major mood episode (depressive or manic) concurrent with Criterion A symptoms of schizophrenia, and at least a two-week period of hallucinations or delusions in the absence of a major mood episode. Hallucinations thus help establish that there is a psychotic process not wholly reducible to mood disturbance, yet the overall course of the illness is dominated by affective episodes. The same hallucinatory content— say, voices commenting on one's actions—would be interpreted differently if it appeared exclusively during severe depression (suggesting a mood disorder with psychotic features) versus occurring both during and outside mood episodes (suggesting schizoaffective disorder). Case-based teaching in psychiatry often turns on such distinctions, inviting trainees to ask not only "what does the patient hear?" but also "when do the voices occur, and in relation to what?" (Malhi et al., 2008).

Mood disorders with psychotic features offer a complementary pattern. In major depressive disorder with psychotic features, DSM-5 specifies that hallucinations or delusions occur only during episodes that otherwise meet full criteria for major depression; once the depressive episode remits, the psychotic symptoms disappear as well. The hallucinations are often mood-congruent: Voices that condemn, accuse or insist on guilt and worthlessness, or somatic hallucinations that echo themes of bodily ruin or disease.

In bipolar I or II disorder with psychotic features, hallucinations occur exclusively in the context of manic, hypomanic or depressive episodes and tend to reflect the prevailing mood state—for example, grandiose voices affirming special powers during euphoric phases or hostile, critical voices in mixed or depressive states. A manic episode is a sustained period of abnormally elevated, expansive or irritable mood accompanied by increased energy or goal-directed activity, often leading to impulsive behaviour, reduced need for sleep, inflated self-esteem and marked impairment in functioning. Bipolar I involves at least one full manic episode, typically more severe and more likely to require hospitalisation, while bipolar II is defined by hypomanic episodes—shorter, less impairing mood elevations—alongside major depressive episodes, without ever reaching full mania. In both forms, when psychotic features appear, they are bound to these mood episodes rather than occurring inde-pendently, making hallucinations an expression of extreme affective states rather than a primary psychotic disorder.

LIVED EXPERIENCE, INSIGHT AND CONTEXT

For people in a psychotic state, hallucinations are rarely just stray sen-sory glitches. They often arrive as fully formed events that demand a response, shaping how a person feels, thinks and relates to others. Auditory verbal hallucinations—especially voices that speak, com-ment or command—are the most common form in schizophrenia spectrum disorders and in mood disorders with psychotic features. Visual hallucinations may accompany them, but large clinical sam-ples suggest that hearing voices is usually the dominant experience in primary psychotic illnesses, with voices perceived as coming from outside the head and carrying a striking sense of agency and intention (McCarthy-Jones et al., 2017). The result is not simply extra noise in consciousness, but a reorganisation of everyday life: Routines gradually bend around the demands or threats of the voices, conversations are interrupted or overshadowed by ongoing commentary and relationships become strained as family and clinicians struggle to understand experiences they cannot share.

Different sensory modalities tend to be associated with different diagnostic patterns, even though there is considerable overlap. In schizophrenia and schizoaffective disorder, auditory hallucinations are particularly characteristic, and they often cluster with delusions of control, thought interference and other disturbances of self-experience. Visual hallucinations in these conditions usually co-occur with voices and other psychotic symptoms, and may take the form of faces, figures or complex scenes that seem embedded in the surrounding world. Tactile phenomena—such as sensations of insects crawling on or under the skin, or of being touched or interfered with—are less common but can be intensely distressing, frequently binding to persecutory or somatic delusions. Olfactory and gustatory hallucinations are rarer in primary psychotic disorders; when smell or taste changes dominate in an otherwise ambiguous picture, clinicians are more likely to consider neurological or medical causes, such as temporal lobe epilepsy, migraine or neurodegenerative disease, before concluding that they are part of a schizophrenia spectrum illness.

Mood disorders with psychotic features display a slightly different configuration of modalities. In major depressive disorder with psychotic features, auditory hallucinations are again common, but they often take on a mood-congruent tone: Voices that condemn, accuse or insist on guilt and worthlessness, sometimes accompanied by somatic hallucinations that echo themes of bodily decay or disease. Bipolar disorder with psychotic features can involve both auditory and visual hallucinations, particularly during manic phases, where voices may praise, encourage or confirm grandiose beliefs, or in mixed states, where voices become hostile or critical. Longitudinal studies suggest that, across schizophrenia, schizoaffective disorder, bipolar disorder and psychotic depression, auditory hallucinations are more frequent than visual ones at baseline and remain more persistent over time, especially in schizophrenia, where both auditory and visual hallucinations tend to be more enduring and multimodal. None of these patterns is absolute, but they guide clinical reasoning: An isolated visual hallucination in an older adult with Parkinson's disease invites a different set of questions than a chorus of talking voices in a young person with disorganised thinking.

The impact of these experiences is shaped not only by their sensory form, but by the person's ability to reflect on them—what clinicians call "insight". Insight is not an all-or-nothing property. It includes several overlapping capacities: Recognising that the experiences are unusual or symptomatic, acknowledging the possibility of having a mental disorder and appreciating the need for treatment or support. Some people insist that what they see or hear is unquestionably real and externally caused, and may reconfigure their lives around these perceptions, avoiding certain places, changing jobs, or breaking relationships in order to escape perceived threats. Others occupy a more ambivalent space, oscillating between conviction and doubt ("it feels real, but I know other people can't hear it"), or adopting a "double bookkeeping" stance in which they act as if both the ordinary world and the hallucinatory world are valid at once. A smaller group can sustain relatively stable insight, recognising their hallucinations as products of the mind even while they are happening, sometimes using this awareness to negotiate or resist the experiences.

Empirical work suggests that poor insight in psychosis is associated with more severe symptoms, greater functional impairment and lower adherence to treatment, whereas better insight often predicts improved clinical and social outcomes, though it can also be linked to increased depression or shame as the person faces the implications of their diagnosis (Lysaker et al., 2018). The degree of insight is not simply a trait; it can fluctuate with stress, mood and the intensity of hallucinations and it is influenced by cultural narratives about what it means to hear voices or see visions. Many people with psychotic disorders move back and forth across the boundary between belief and scepticism, sometimes within the same day and their distress often depends less on the sensory vividness of the hallucinations than on how much room they feel they have to question, reinterpret or live alongside them.

The developmental and social context in which hallucinations emerge plays a crucial role in how they are experienced and understood. Childhood trauma, bullying and social adversity have been shown to increase the likelihood of later hallucinatory experiences (Shevlin et al., 2007), and these histories can leave their imprint on content: Voices may echo themes of threat, humiliation or abandonment drawn from earlier relationships. Adolescents who begin to hear voices or see figures often do so against a background of other subtle changes—heightened self-consciousness, unusual perceptual sensitivities or a sense that thoughts are no longer entirely private—which phenomenological approaches describe as a gradual transformation of the "field" of consciousness rather than a sudden intrusion of isolated hallucinations. For some, these experiences remain intermittent and are integrated into a relatively stable sense of self; for others, they progressively erode confidence in their own perceptions, leading to social withdrawal, fear of "going mad" and breakdowns in education or work.

Culture and social environment, in turn, provide the language and frameworks through which hallucinations are interpreted. Comparative studies of voice-hearers in different countries, for instance, find that people in some non-Western settings are more likely to describe their voices as more pleasant, while Western clinical populations more often report hostile or persecutory voices, a difference that appears to reflect broader cultural scripts about spirits, illness and selfhood (Khaled et al., 2023). One of the best-known examples is Tanya Luhrmann's comparative work with people diagnosed with schizophrenia in the United States, Ghana and India (Luhrmann et al., 2015). In a sample of 60 participants (20 in each site), her team found that American participants tended to describe their voices as intrusive, harsh and violent, experienced as symptoms of a diseased mind, whereas many Ghanaian and Indian participants reported more benign, playful or relational voices, sometimes interpreted as spirits or deities.

Within any given culture, subgroups offer alternative ways of narrating psychotic experiences, sometimes encouraging a view of voices as meaningful or as aspects of the self, rather than as purely pathological phenomena. Such contexts can bolster insight in a nuanced sense: A person may come to see their hallucinations as real experiences with psychological or spiritual significance, while also recognising that the literal claims made by the voices (e.g., "you are evil", "everyone hates you") need not be accepted at face value. In this way, lived experience, insight and context interweave: What is heard or seen, what diagnosis is given, how real it feels and how liveable it becomes all depend on the intricate interplay between the brain's generative machinery, the person's developmental history and the social worlds that receive—or refuse—their testimony.

HALLUCINATIONS, RISK AND THE STORIES PEOPLE TELL

When hallucinations occur in psychosis, they often extend beyond mere commentary and enter the realm of command. A voice might instruct someone to cut themselves, jump, or attack another person. Because such "command hallucinations" appear to link symptoms with action, they dominate public fears about psychosis. Yet clinical and first-person accounts reveal that risk rarely follows such direct lines (Birchwood et al., 2014). Many people negotiate with their voices—arguing, delaying or ignoring orders for years. Their stories expose a far more intricate web of influences than the command alone.

Consider a young man in his early twenties facing his first episode of psychosis. For months, he has heard a male voice critical and accusatory, sometimes challenging him to "prove your strength" by cutting his arms. Most days he resists, distracting himself with music, pacing, or calling a friend until the command fades. After an explosive argument at home, however, he complies, inflicting shallow cuts that alarm him the moment he sees blood. In the emergency department he says, "The voice made me do it", describing an encounter in which the voice feels like an external agent and his own will disappears.

Later, when calm returns, his story expands. He remembers earlier thoughts of self-harm, feelings of entrapment and humiliation and an unspoken hope that visible wounds might communicate distress he could not otherwise express. The voice remains important, but now exists within a broader field of despair, anger and unmet needs. Risk becomes understandable not as a simple reaction to hallucinated orders, but as the intersection of strong emotions, meaning and circumstance. The shift from "the voice controlled me" to "the voice and everything else overwhelmed me" captures how people reconstruct agency once the crisis has passed.

Empirical studies mirror this complexity (Hersh & Borum, 1998). Those who experience violent or self-destructive commands do show higher rates of such behaviour than people whose voices merely comment or converse—especially when the voice is perceived as powerful, knowing or protective. Yet most individuals resist complying. When they do, their actions often align with existing emotional states: Suicidal commands during depression, aggressive commands during fear or rage. The content of the hallucination interacts with hopelessness, impulsivity, substance use, access to means and social context. Words alone do not dictate behaviour; they meet the person in a particular psychological and situational landscape.

Acts of violence attributed to psychosis tell similar stories of convergence. A woman with long-term schizophrenia might push a stranger, later explaining that she believed he was the assassin from her recurring visions. What seems random from outside appears to her as pre-emptive self-defence, a desperate response to threat. Later, she recalls a flicker of doubt even as she acted—an instant of awareness that things might not be real—showing that agency can persist even within delusion and fear.

How others respond to such crises profoundly shapes later narratives. When family or clinicians focus only on danger—"Your voices make you unsafe"—people may learn that disclosure invites condemnation and retreat into silence. More curious, empathic responses—asking what the voice said, how it felt, what else was happening—invite richer accounts where hallucinations are potent but not omnipotent. In these contexts, individuals begin to recognise points of hesitation and choice, reframing their experiences as battles within the self rather than total surrender to madness.

Autobiographical accounts often trace a movement from stories of compulsion to those of shared influence. Early on, people may declare, "The voices control me; I'm dangerous". Gradually, some come to recognise patterns: "They're strongest when I'm tired or alone. Sometimes I can resist". The transformation seen in memoirs such as Elyn Saks's (2007) *The Center Cannot Hold* vividly reflects this journey—Saks describes how voices that once dictated her actions became experiences she could observe, challenge and to some degree manage once understanding replaced fear. Hallucinations remain frightening, but they no longer define the person's entire moral identity. Episodes once seen as proof of inherent danger can later be understood as outcomes of combined illness, stress and circumstance—a voice speaking despair that had long been building.

Crucially, these personal and clinical stories reshape future experience. Someone who now interprets command hallucinations as warning signs rather than orders may reach out for support instead of acting. Another may notice their voices worsen when physically run-down or under strain and begin to treat those states as part of the risk, not background noise. Through such reinterpretations, narrative itself becomes therapeutic: Turning moments of horror into integrated parts of an ongoing life, where meaning and control can coexist with symptoms.

This exploration of how people make sense of psychosis points towards a broader question: What happens when hallucinatory worlds emerge not only from psychiatric illness but from neurological disturbance or sensory deprivation? The next chapter follows this transition—from voices and visions embedded in the dramas of self and story, to those arising from the body and brain in conditions such as Parkinson's disease, epilepsy, migraine and delirium.

4

HALLUCINATIONS IN NEUROLOGICAL AND MEDICAL CONDITIONS

In 1817, the English surgeon James Parkinson published *An Essay on the Shaking Palsy*, a slim pamphlet that would later give its author's name to a whole neurodegenerative disorder. He described tremor, stiffness and slowness of movement in six patients he had observed on the streets of London, noting how their bodies betrayed them while their minds appeared "uninjured" (Parkinson, 1817). What he did not describe were the strangers some of these patients would one day come to see sitting in their living rooms, or the small animals darting at the edges of their vision, long after the tremor began.

Nearly two centuries later, neurologists started to realise that the "shaking palsy" was accompanied, for many people, by a much quieter but equally striking symptom: visual hallucinations (Fénelon et al., 2000). Patients who had once fit Parkinson's image of an intact mind in a failing body began to report seeing children playing in the hallway when no one was there, or groups of unfamiliar people standing in the corner of the room, watching silently. Some saw cats or dogs that slipped away when the light was switched on; others saw intricate patterns or shadowy figures that faded when they tried to look directly at them. At first, these experiences were dismissed as "side effects" of medications, or as signs of depression or dementia,

DOI: 10.4324/9781003784890-5

but large clinical studies gradually made clear that hallucinations are woven into the natural history of Parkinson's disease itself.

It is estimated that up to half of people living with Parkinson's disease will experience hallucinations or related psychotic symptoms at some point in the course of their illness, especially in later stages (Aarsland et al., 1999). These are most often visual, but can also involve other senses. Many patients retain at least partial insight, recognising that what they see is "not quite real", while others become convinced and frightened, insisting that strangers are entering the house or that insects infest the walls. For years, however, such experiences went largely unspoken in neurology clinics: patients feared being labelled "crazy", families did not know how to bring the topic up and clinicians focused on motor symptoms that were easier to measure.

This chapter begins from that historical blind spot and widens it. Its focus is on hallucinations that arise primarily in neurological and general medical conditions—Parkinson's disease and dementia with Lewy bodies, epilepsies, migraine aura, structural brain disease, sensory loss and acute medical or surgical states. In these contexts, something is happening to the brain or body that reshapes perception from the outside in: dopamine pathways are altered, sensory input is degraded, cortical networks are disturbed by seizures or inflammation, or the whole system is pushed into a metabolic or infectious crisis. The hallucinations that follow are not incidental curiosities; they are part of how illnesses manifest themselves in lived experience.

Despite their clinical importance, such hallucinations are often under-recognised outside psychiatry. Delirium—an acute disturbance of attention and awareness, frequently accompanied by vivid visual hallucinations—occurs in a substantial proportion of hospitalised patients, particularly older adults and those in intensive care, yet is still missed or misdiagnosed in many cases, with direct consequences for treatment decisions, safety and length of stay. People with Parkinson's disease may quietly navigate around hallucinated animals or speak in lowered tones about "visitors" they know others cannot see, while consultations revolve around medication schedules and gait, and individuals with severe visual loss may endure months of silent, complex visions before anyone names what is happening to them. Patients emerging from intensive care unit (ICU) may carry disturbing memories of spiders on the ceiling or masked figures at the bedside without realising these were delirium-related hallucinations shared by many others, and their families are left to manage fear, confusion and practical risks at home. Precisely because these experiences sit at the intersection of neurology, general medicine and mental health, studying them is crucial: they reveal how specific brain and body changes distort perception, refine broader theories of how the mind constructs reality and highlight concrete opportunities for clinicians to recognise, explain and address hallucinations in the settings where they most often remain invisible.

HALLUCINATIONS IN NEUROLOGICAL DISORDERS

Hallucinations in neurological disorders often have a distinctive pattern that sets them apart from those associated with primary psychotic illnesses. In conditions such as Parkinson's disease, dementia with Lewy bodies, epilepsy, migraine and structural brain disease, hallucinations tend to follow the contours of the underlying brain changes: their timing, sensory modality and degree of insight are closely tied to particular networks being disrupted rather than to a global breakdown of reality-testing.

Parkinson's disease is usually known as a movement disorder: It causes tremor, stiffness and slowness because the brain cells that produce the chemical messenger dopamine gradually die off. Yet many people with Parkinson's also develop changes in perception, including vivid hallucinations that are now seen as part of a broader "Parkinson's psychosis" rather than a rare side-effect tagged onto the motor symptoms (Fénelon & Alves, 2010). As people live longer with the condition and receive effective dopamine-based medications, a sizeable minority begin to see things that are not there, often in otherwise ordinary settings like their living rooms or bedrooms. These experiences often start quietly, with a fleeting sense that someone has just walked past the doorway, or that a cat or dog has slipped by at the edge of vision, only to vanish when the person turns their head. Over time, these brief impressions can develop into clear, detailed images of people, children or animals, usually appearing in familiar places and often simply sitting or standing nearby, present but not interacting.

The celebrated neurologist Oliver Sacks (2013, ch. 5) describes one such case from his clinical experience: "Ed W., a designer, started to get visual hallucinations after he had been on L-dopa and dopamine agonists for several years. He realised that they were hallucinations and regarded them largely with curiosity and amusement. ... He started to have hallucinations of people who entered his apartment, emerging from "a secret chamber" behind the kitchen. "They invade my privacy", Ed said. "They occupy my space. ... They are very interested in me—they take notes, take photos, rifle through my papers". Sometimes they had sex—one of the intruders was a very beautiful woman, and sometimes three or four of them would occupy Ed's bed when he was not using it".

In the earlier stages, many people realise that these figures cannot be real, even though they look uncannily lifelike; later on, especially if memory and thinking also worsen, the same figures may be treated as genuine visitors or intruders, leading to fear, checking behaviours or clashes with relatives who see nothing at all. Medication is part of the story but not the whole of it: Drugs such as levodopa and dopamine agonists improve movement but also raise the risk of visual hallucinations (Friedman, 1991), particularly at higher doses and over longer periods, so that adjusting the prescription can sometimes reduce the problem at the price of stiffer, slower movement. In other cases, hallucinations continue despite careful dose reduction, suggesting that changes in the brain's visual and attention systems—shaped by the disease itself and by other transmitters such as acetylcholine—also play a key role in shifting perception away from the outside world and towards internally generated images.

Dementia with Lewy bodies is a form of dementia that affects thinking, movement, sleep and perception, named after tiny abnormal clumps of protein ("Lewy bodies") that build up inside nerve cells in key brain regions. Like Alzheimer's disease, it causes problems with memory and everyday cognition, but it is particularly marked by a combination of fluctuating attention, Parkinson's-like motor symptoms (such as stiffness and slowness), disturbances of sleep in which people may act out their dreams, and recurrent, well-formed visual hallucinations. People often describe seeing people, animals or small creatures in ordinary settings, with striking clarity and detail.

Unlike in Parkinson's disease, where hallucinations were long assumed to be mainly a side-effect of medication, in Lewy body dementia, these visions commonly appear early on, sometimes even before the movement problems are obvious, and can therefore be an important early clue that this particular type of dementia is developing (Onofrj et al., 2013). How people relate to these experiences varies greatly: Some quickly recognise that the vivid figures they see are "tricks of the mind", while others treat them as part of everyday reality, chatting to invisible visitors or quietly laying out extra plates and cups for guests that family members cannot see. A hallmark of the condition is fluctuation: Concentration and alertness can change markedly over hours or days, with hallucinations becoming more frequent and intense when the person is drowsy, confused or "foggy", then fading when they are more alert and clear-headed.

As Lewy bodies spread through visual and related networks, particularly in regions that help the brain organise and interpret what the eyes see, the visual system seems more likely to fill in gaps by generating convincing people and objects whenever incoming information is ambiguous, especially in dim lighting, when the person is tired, or under stress. In clinical practice, this pattern—recurrent, detailed visual hallucinations in an older adult, together with fluctuating cognition and mild Parkinson-like signs—is more suggestive of a Lewy body process than of a primary psychiatric psychosis, and it has important treatment implications, since standard antipsychotic drugs can trigger severe worsening of movement and even serious medical complications in this group and must therefore be used, if at all, with extreme caution.

Likewise, epilepsy brings with it a distinctive style of hallucinatory experience, usually packed into very short bursts and closely linked to where in the brain the seizure begins (Kasper et al., 2010). In focal epilepsy—especially when seizures originate in the temporal or occipital lobes—people often experience a warning or "aura" before the main episode (Jaballah et al., 2022). This aura can include vivid lights, voices, smells or even a fleeting sense of being transported into another scene. Such experiences are characteristically repetitive: The same coloured patch in the same visual field, the same tune or odour, or an identical surge of familiarity before the seizure returns—like the brain replaying an internal clip. The Russian novelist Fyodor Dostoevsky famously described such moments, recalling in his temporal lobe epilepsy an overwhelming flash of joy and revelation seconds before losing consciousness, which he considered both ecstatic and terrifying (Seneviratne, 2010). Visual experiences linked to occipital seizures have their own distinct flavour, helping to differentiate them from migraine aura or psychotic visions. These typically appear as brief, brightly coloured geometric forms that move or "march" across the field of view, flickering on and off abruptly with mechanical precision (Cowan, 2015).

In some forms of occipital epilepsy, visual hallucinations can grow complex, unfolding as shifting scenes or animated figures. Yet the crucial feature is their tight link to other seizure markers—forced eye movements, automatisms or a rapid plunge into altered consciousness. These are contained, time-bounded events rather than parallel realities coexisting with daily life. When seizures originate in the temporal lobes, the experiences can be especially striking, involving voices, melodies or emotionally saturated scenes that might superficially resemble psychotic symptoms. A well-known example is that of composer Robert Schumann, who, during probable focal seizures, described hearing entire orchestral passages and celestial choirs, sounds that later intertwined with his creative work but also heralded his neurological and psychiatric decline (Ostwald, 1985). Even in such cases, the defining pattern remains brevity and recurrence: Hallucinations repeat in nearly identical form, last only seconds or minutes and leave the person dazed or amnesic—very different from the variable, prolonged hallucinatory episodes common in schizophrenia or severe mood disorders.

Migraine—a common neurological condition in which people have recurrent attacks of headache and nausea—brings a different kind of brief disturbance to the visual world, especially when it occurs with aura (Schott, 2007). In this form, people often describe luminous zigzag lines, shimmering castle-like patterns or expanding blind spots that slowly drift across their field of vision over 10–30 minutes, sometimes accompanied by flickering geometric shapes or odd changes in how big or small things look. These visual effects usually involve both eyes, follow a fairly similar script each time for a given person, and unfold gradually rather than appearing and disappearing in an instant; they are often followed by headache, nausea and sensitivity to light and sound, though some people experience the aura without any pain at all.

Compared with the visual hallucinations that can occur in epilepsy, migraine auras are typically less colourful and more black-and-white or high-contrast, more jagged or linear, and slower to spread, reflecting a different underlying process in the brain. Crucially, most people remain fully aware that something is wrong with their vision, pause activities such as driving, and trust that the disturbance will fade within a familiar time window. Fully formed people or objects very rarely appear in migraine aura; if they do, or if the aura lasts unusually long or comes with atypical symptoms, clinicians are more likely to consider additional causes such as coexisting epilepsy or a structural brain problem and to investigate further (Hartl et al., 2017).

Structural problems in the brain—such as strokes, tumours or areas of local shrinkage—can also give rise to hallucinations, and these tend to be brief, localised and surprisingly informative about where the damage is. Lesions in the occipital lobes, which are heavily involved in vision, may produce simple visual hallucinations restricted to one part of the visual field, sometimes only on one side, whereas damage in parietal or temporal regions can layer in more complex shapes, faces or even short scene-like images (Anderson & Rizzo, 1994). In contrast to the more diffuse, multi-sensory hallucinations that can appear in a psychotic episode, these lesion-related experiences often behave almost like a neurological sign: The same corner of the visual world repeatedly sprouts colours or patterns, or the same type of image recurs alongside other local problems such as weakness, numbness or difficulties with speech. Although they can be distressing, their pattern usually stays closely tied to the underlying anatomy and blood supply, and they seldom grow into elaborate stories of persecution or complex delusional systems unless wider networks responsible for belief-formation and sense of self are also affected.

HALLUCINATIONS IN SENSORY LOSS AND ACUTE MEDICAL STATES

Hallucinations do not only arise in long-standing brain disorders like Parkinson's disease or epilepsy. They also appear in situations where the senses are deprived of input, or where the body is acutely unwell and the brain is struggling to maintain a coherent grip on the environment (Fénelon, 2013). In these contexts, the experiences can be extraordinarily vivid and convincing, yet they often follow patterns quite different from those seen in psychotic illnesses. They tend to be closely tied to the state of the sensory organs or to temporary disturbances in attention, metabolism or consciousness.

One of the clearest examples of hallucinations driven by sensory loss is Charles Bonnet syndrome. As mentioned in Chapter 2, this term refers to complex visual hallucinations that occur in people with significant loss of sight, typically due to conditions such as macular degeneration, glaucoma or diabetic eye disease, who are otherwise mentally well. A person may have poor vision or large blind spots when tested, yet report seeing detailed images of people, animals, patterns or entire scenes. The content can be remarkably elaborate: Tiny, vividly dressed figures marching across the floor, faces that appear over wallpaper, or intricate geometric designs overlaying walls and ceilings. Importantly, these images are projected into the external space, like ordinary perception, not just "seen in the mind's eye". And yet insight is often preserved: Many people know, or quickly come to suspect, that what they are seeing cannot be real, especially when family members confirm that they see nothing unusual.

From a psychological and neurological perspective, Charles Bonnet syndrome is often described as an example of "release" hallucinations (Kelson et al., 2022). The idea is that when normal visual input is reduced or lost—because the retina no longer sends a rich stream of information to the brain—the visual cortex is no longer held in check by the outside world. Deprived of its usual workload, it begins to fire spontaneously and to generate its own images, drawing on memory, pattern-detection and the brain's tendency to make sense of noise. In this view, the hallucinations are not signs of a mind unhinged, but of visual pathways that are suddenly under-constrained: they are released to create. The fact that many people with Charles Bonnet syndrome retain insight fits with this picture. Their higher-level thinking, memory and sense of reality remain intact; what has changed is the reliability of the visual feed reaching those cognitive systems.

These sensory-deprivation phenomena sit at one end of a spectrum in which hallucinations are driven as much by what is missing from perception as by what is present. At the other end are acute medical and surgical states, where the problem is less about loss of input and more about a general disruption of how the brain organises and filters information. Delirium is the classic example. Rather than being a disease in itself, delirium is a syndrome—a pattern of changes in attention, awareness and thinking—that can be triggered by many underlying causes: infections, high fevers, metabolic imbalances, drug toxicity, alcohol withdrawal, surgery, organ failure and more. People in delirium are characteristically disoriented and distractible, their level of alertness waxing and waning over hours. Within that shifting state, hallucinations are common, often blending into illusions and misinterpretations of the environment (Tachibana et al., 2021).

The hallucinations of delirium can be dramatic. A hospital room may be transformed into a battlefield or a childhood home. Ordinary staff and relatives may be perceived as strangers, invaders or religious figures. Small animals, insects or shadowy figures may be seen moving across the bed or walls. Auditory experiences can range from indistinct mumbling or music to clear voices calling the person's name or issuing commands. Crucially, these experiences are tightly bound to the disturbance in attention and consciousness: When the delirium lifts and orientation returns, the hallucinations usually fade or vanish altogether. In contrast to the often enduring, self-consistent voices or visions in chronic psychosis, delirious hallucinations tend to be fragmented, fluctuating and influenced by the immediate environment—for example, patterns in curtains, flickering lights or snippets of overheard conversation.

ICUs provide a particularly striking setting for such experiences (Hall et al., 2012). Patients there are often critically ill, attached to machines, sedated, sleep-deprived and surrounded by unfamiliar sounds and alarms. In this context, hallucinations and delusion-like ideas are extremely common. A person may be convinced that staff is plotting to harm them, that wires and tubes are snakes, or that they are being held captive in a submarine, factory or prison. These beliefs and perceptions can persist in memory long after discharge, contributing to post-traumatic stress symptoms. The combination of sensory overload (constant noise, invasive procedures) and sensory deprivation (no natural daylight, restricted movement, disrupted sleep) creates a fertile ground for the brain to generate threatening narratives to make sense of an otherwise incomprehensible situation.

More broadly, acute disturbances in the body's chemistry can also provoke transient hallucinations (Bonnot et al., 2015). Sudden swings in blood sugar, severe liver or kidney failure with toxin build-up, low oxygen, high carbon dioxide or systemic infections can all affect how brain cells function. The result may be a picture in which hallucinations, confusion, fluctuating attention and emotional lability appear together and resolve once the underlying medical problem is addressed.

A key feature linking these acute medical states is their time course and reversibility. While the experiences can be terrifying and may leave emotional scars, they are typically confined to the period when the body and brain are under acute strain. As the infection is controlled, the metabolic imbalance corrected, or the sedative levels reduced, the person gradually regains the ability to focus, track conversations and distinguish dreams from reality, and the hallucinations subside. This temporal link is diagnostically important. It directs clinicians to search for medical triggers—checking vital signs, blood tests, medication lists and signs of withdrawal—rather than treating the hallucinations purely as a psychiatric episode.

Across these neurological and medical settings, a shared theme is that hallucinations tend to appear where perception is under pressure rather than because there is a single "madness centre" in the mind. The brain keeps trying to do its usual job—building a workable picture of the world from the signals it receives—but in Parkinson's disease, Lewy body dementia, epilepsy, migraine, visual loss and delirium, that job is being done on shaky ground, with damaged pathways, missing information or organs in crisis. In those conditions, extra figures, scenes and voices often slip into the picture as the system improvises with whatever it has. What sets these hallucinations apart from those in primary psychotic disorders is not that they feel less real, but that their style and timing track particular changes in vision, attention, arousal or bodily chemistry and often fade as those underlying problems improve. The next chapter follows this idea into another in-between zone: sleep. There, as the brain moves in and out of dreaming and different sleep stages, the border between waking and sleeping can blur and hallucination-like experiences may appear at the edges of sleep—just as we are drifting off or starting to wake—offering another way to see how small shifts in brain state can change the line between what is perceived and what is imagined.

5

HALLUCINATIONS AND SLEEP

In 1846, the French psychiatrist Jules Baillarger published *On the influence of the intermediate state between waking and sleeping on the production and course of hallucinations*. He wrote about patients who, just as they were drifting off or about to wake up, suddenly saw vivid figures and scenes that vanished moments later (Blom, 2023). What struck him was not only how strange these visions were, but when they appeared: In those unstable moments between waking and sleeping, when the mind is neither fully on nor fully off and perception loosens its usual grip on reality. People described landscapes, faces, voices and a sense of presence that felt as real as anything they encountered while awake, yet had no clear source and disappeared as quickly as they came. These early reports suggested that the in-between zones of sleep might be especially fertile ground for hallucinatory experiences.

Most people are familiar with the idea that dreams are "like hallucinations", rich internal dramas generated while the body lies still in bed, but for many, the most unsettling experiences associated with sleep occur just before drifting off or just after waking. A person may hear their name called in an empty room, or awaken to the unmistakable sensation that someone is standing at the foot of the

DOI: 10.4324/9781003784890-6

bed, watching. For a few seconds, the experience is utterly convincing; only later does doubt creep in. These episodes can be startling or terrifying, yet they are not necessarily signs of madness or brain disease. Instead, they grow out of the ordinary physiology of sleep and waking, and of the delicate choreography that normally keeps perception, dreaming and bodily control aligned.

This chapter explores what happens when that choreography slips. It focuses on hallucinations that occur in the context of sleep and its disturbances: The fleeting images and sounds of hypnagogic (falling-asleep) and hypnopompic (waking-up) states, the frightening visions and bodily sensations that accompany sleep paralysis and the complex experiences that arise in conditions such as narcolepsy and certain parasomnias. When people hallucinate in association with sleep, the experiences arise at predictable points in the sleep–wake cycle and often in otherwise healthy individuals, making them a valuable test case for understanding how changes in arousal and attention can generate perception-like experiences in the absence of appropriate external input.

During normal sleep, the brain and body pass through a repeating pattern of stages, from light drowsiness to deep, slow-wave sleep and into rapid eye movement (REM) sleep, when dreaming is most intense (Hobson, 2009). In waking life, brain activity, muscle tone and responsiveness to the environment usually align; in certain sleep-related hallucinations, by contrast, elements of different states are misaligned. A person may be cognitively awake enough to register their surroundings but still caught in REM-like paralysis, or may find fragments of dream imagery "leaking" into a state they experience as waking. The result is a hybrid condition in which the mind treats internally generated content as if it were part of the external here-and-now.

Because these experiences are common, they invite a more graded view of where "normal" ends and "abnormal" begins. Many people will, at some point, see a fleeting figure while drifting off, hear a loud bang that has no source, or feel a presence in the room as they awaken, yet never seek psychiatric care. For others, especially those with narcolepsy or chronic sleep disruption, such episodes can be frequent and distressing, interfering with daily functioning and feeding fears of losing one's mind. The same basic mechanisms—instability at the sleep–wake boundary, partial intrusion of dream states into waking, mismatches between bodily paralysis and a sense of alertness—can underpin both benign and clinically significant experiences, echoing the broader continuum of hallucinations described earlier in the book.

SLEEP ARCHITECTURE AND THE HALLUCINATORY THRESHOLD

Sleep does not simply switch on and off. It arrives in a series of changing brain and body states that cycle several times each night, and in some of those delicate in-between moments, the usual coordination between perception, muscle tone and awareness loosens, leaving small openings through which hallucination-like experiences can slip. Over a typical night, sleep runs in cycles of about 90–110 minutes, each one moving through non-rapid eye movement (NREM) sleep, then REM sleep, before drifting back towards wakefulness. NREM is not just one state but a gradual slide from light drowsiness into deep, slow-wave sleep, during which brain activity becomes more synchronised and the sleeper grows less responsive to sounds, touches and other external events. REM sleep is almost the mirror opposite: The brain becomes highly active and generates rich internal activity, while the body is held in near-complete paralysis by brainstem systems that temporarily shut down most voluntary muscles (Le Bon, 2020).

From the outside, sleep seems to follow a neat, repeating pattern, but from the inside, it feels more changeable and uneven. As wakefulness gives way to light non-REM sleep, attention drifts, thoughts blur and mental images become looser and more picture-like. Later in the night, REM periods usually lengthen and bunch together towards morning, which is why the final hours of sleep so often contain vivid, story-like dreams. Still, these cycles are not rigid.

They are continually shaped by the circadian system—the brain's roughly 24-hour clock—and by homeostatic sleep pressure, the growing "need for sleep", the longer someone stays awake. Together, these processes nudge the brain towards sleep at some times and wakefulness at others, and in doing so help decide when the delicate border zones around sleep, where perception is most likely to wobble, will be crossed.

Under this familiar pattern of sleep cycles sits a busy control system that decides whether the brain tilts towards being awake, deeply asleep or somewhere in between. Key regions in the brainstem and hypothalamus—such as the reticular formation, locus coeruleus, dorsal raphe and clusters of orexin-producing cells—broadcast chemical signals using neuromodulators like acetylcholine, norepinephrine, serotonin, histamine and orexin to set overall levels of alertness. When these systems fire strongly, the cortex is switched "on" and becomes responsive to the outside world; when they quiet down, the brain shifts into NREM sleep, with its typical dampening of responses to sounds, touches and other stimuli.

At the same time, the brain is not simply letting sensory information pour in unfiltered: The thalamus, often called the brain's relay station, decides which sensory signals reach the cortex and how strongly they are represented, changing its firing style across sleep and wake. During deep NREM sleep, thalamic neurons fire in rhythmic bursts that interrupt the smooth relay of outside input, reinforcing the feeling of being shut off from the environment, whereas in wakefulness, the thalamus supports a more continuous flow of information, allowing sights, sounds and other sensations to keep perception firmly tied to what is actually happening around us. REM sleep complicates things again, because in REM the cortex is highly active and driven largely by internal signals while the thalamus continues to restrict much of the external input, so that the dream world can unfold with relatively little interference from real events in the bedroom. This unusual pairing—strong internal activation combined with partial sensory shutdown—helps explain why dream images and sounds can feel as vivid and immediate as waking perception, yet remain largely insulated from what is going on in the outside world.

The most fertile ground for sleep-related hallucinations lies in the narrow moments when REM sleep brushes up against waking. During a typical REM phase, the brainstem switches on muscle atonia, a near-total paralysis of most voluntary muscles, while at the same time driving the REMs and heightened cortical activity that go with dreaming. Normally, these features stay neatly bundled together inside sleep: The person is unaware of the bedroom, unable to move and fully absorbed in an inner world that will later be recognised as a dream. But this coordination is not perfect. At times, elements of REM physiology leak into states the person experiences as being awake or almost awake. In these moments, someone may be clearly aware of lying in bed, able to take in the layout of the room and even hear sounds from outside, yet still find that vivid, dream-like images and sensations pour into consciousness.

Muscle atonia can linger in this state, leaving the person unable to move or call out, even as the mind insists that a figure is standing by the bed or that some presence has entered the room. In the opposite direction, as sleep is beginning, fragments of dream imagery can appear while the person still feels partially awake and able to observe their own thoughts. In both directions—drifting into sleep and rising out of it—the brain passes through brief corridors where features of wakefulness and REM dreaming overlap, creating conditions in which internally generated scenes can feel as if they are happening here and now.

Several aspects of these in-between states make hallucination-like experiences more likely. As people drift towards sleep, it becomes harder to hold steady, reality-testing thoughts; attention starts to fragment, and spontaneous images, sounds or ideas are less likely to be questioned or pushed aside. The brain also loosens its standards for what counts as a plausible event, becoming more accepting of sudden scene changes, odd juxtapositions and gaps that would normally trigger doubt. At the same time, chemical shifts in neuromodulators—especially changes in cholinergic and monoaminergic activity around the start and end of REM—tilt the balance away from sensory-driven processing and towards internally generated activity. Together, these changes create a mental environment in which a fleeting image, a random noise or a brief sense that "someone is there" can catch hold and quickly swell into a vivid experience. This threshold is not fixed for everyone. Differences in how people regulate arousal, cope with stress and recover from lost sleep all affect how smoothly the brain moves across the borders of sleep. Those who are chronically sleep-deprived, highly stressed or subject to irregular sleep schedules often find that the edges of sleep become frayed—slipping in and out of light sleep, waking more often from REM or spending longer in mixed, intermediate states.

HYPNAGOGIC AND HYPNOPOMPIC HALLUCINATIONS

Hypnagogic and hypnopompic hallucinations sit in the thin borderlands between waking and sleep, when the mind is neither fully anchored in the outside world nor fully surrendered to dreaming (Waters et al., 2016). Hypnagogic experiences arise as a person drifts off, in the minutes when eyelids droop, thoughts loosen and sleep has not yet fully taken hold. Hypnopompic experiences appear on the way back, as consciousness is returning and the sleeper is surfacing towards wakefulness. In both directions, perception becomes unusually labile. The brain momentarily treats its own internally generated images, sounds and sensations as if they were happening in the bedroom, producing experiences that can be as vivid as anything in daytime life, yet last only seconds or a minute or two before dissolving.

The most common form of these borderland experiences is visual (Waters et al., 2024). Someone lying in bed may suddenly "see" a figure standing in the doorway, a person sitting at the bedside or a small animal on the pillow, often in sharp detail and with a sense of presence that is hard to dismiss in the moment. Another person might watch geometric patterns, flashes of light or rapidly shifting landscapes unfold behind closed eyes, as if a private cinema had been switched on just as they were falling asleep. These images tend to be brief and unstable. Many people describe them as startling rather than deeply terrifying, especially when they occur only once in a while and are recognised, in hindsight, as "just something that happens when I'm very tired".

Auditory experiences are also common. Instead of a coherent conversation or sustained voice, people often report hearing their own name called, a single word spoken sharply in their ear, or a brief phrase that has no obvious source. Others describe hearing a door slam, glass shatter, a loud bang inside the head or a short burst of music that stops as soon as they fully awaken. In a typical vignette, a student who has been working late finally lies down, hovers in that half-asleep state and suddenly hears a clear male voice say "Hey!" from just beside the bed. Heart racing, she sits up, turns on the light and finds no one there. Once the initial fear passes, she realises that the voice coincided exactly with the moment she was tipping into sleep. The next day, she may recount it as strange but not life-changing, perhaps even slightly amusing.

Tactile and body-related sensations add another layer (Cheyne, 2003). Some people feel a light touch on the arm, a pressure on the chest or the distinct impression that the mattress is dipping as if someone has just sat down. Others report tingling, vibrations or a sense that the body is stretching, shrinking or levitating. These experiences can be deeply uncanny because they recruit the internal map of the body in space. A man might drift off and suddenly feel as if his legs are floating upwards while his torso remains on the bed, or as if the whole bed is tilting sideways or spinning gently. These vestibular sensations—linked to the systems that normally register balance and motion—can make the room seem to sway or rotate even though everything is still. The person may open their eyes to check, and for a heartbeat, the mismatch between what they feel and what they see further amplifies the sense of unreality.

Perhaps the most unsettling, and yet very common, feature of these experiences is the feeling that someone or something is present.

This "presence" sensation does not always come with a clear image. A person waking in the dark might feel an intense certainty that another being is in the room, just out of sight, watching, approaching or looming near the bed. Sometimes this presence is vaguely defined; at other times it is immediately labelled—a stranger, an intruder, a supernatural figure.

Despite how intense they can feel, these hypnagogic and hypnopompic hallucinations are usually brief, self-limited and surprisingly common in the general population. Many large surveys suggest that a significant minority of people have had at least one such episode in their lives, often in periods of sleep deprivation, jet lag, stress or irregular schedules (Ohayon et al., 1996). For most, these experiences remain rare curiosities. Crucially, once fully awake, people typically regain insight. They may not have been sure at the time whether the figure or voice was real, but in the cold light of morning, they reclassify the event as something that "must have been my mind" rather than evidence that the bedroom was genuinely occupied.

Comparing them with ordinary dreams helps sharpen the picture. Dreams usually unfold within sustained sleep, especially during REM, and they are embedded in a continuous narrative world that feels normal while it lasts. The dreamer rarely questions whether they are dreaming; the absurdities of the dream environment are accepted as given. Only on awakening does the person step back, recognise discontinuities and reclassify the entire episode as unreal. Hypnagogic and hypnopompic hallucinations, by contrast, occur at the edges of sleep, when the person feels at least partly awake and still anchored in the actual bedroom. The dream-like content erupts into what is experienced as the real here-and-now environment. Rather than being absorbed into a long story, the experience often takes the form of a single, striking event: one figure, one voice, one startling sensation.

They also differ in important ways from daytime hallucinations associated with psychosis or neurological disease. As we have already seen, hallucinations in conditions such as schizophrenia,

Parkinson's disease or certain forms of epilepsy typically appear during stable waking consciousness. The person is clearly awake, engaged in daytime activities and the hallucinations recur or persist, often in multiple contexts; these experiences are not confined to the fragile boundaries of sleep and are usually part of a broader clinical picture that includes changes in mood, thinking, behaviour or neurological functioning. By contrast, a hypnagogic hallucination that occurs once a month when someone is exhausted, lasts a few seconds and is later recognised as sleep-related does not, on its own, indicate psychosis.

SLEEP PARALYSIS, NARCOLEPSY AND PARASOMNIAS

Sleep paralysis is perhaps the clearest example of what happens when REM sleep does not stay neatly in its allotted box (D'Agostino & Limosani, 2010). In REM, as earlier sections have shown, the brain normally generates vivid internal imagery while the body is held in near-total paralysis, preventing dream movements from being acted out. In sleep paralysis, this paralysis leaks into a state that feels subjectively awake. A person opens their eyes, registers the familiar contours of their bedroom, hears traffic or the hum of a fan and yet finds that no matter how desperately they try, they cannot move a finger or force a sound out of their throat. The basic perceptions of the room are real, but they are overlaid with an intense sense of vulnerability produced by the mismatch between a seemingly awake mind and an unresponsive body.

This mismatch lays the groundwork for characteristic hallucinations. One common pattern is a felt presence. Another is pressure on the chest, described as a weight, a person sitting or kneeling on the torso, or an invisible force pinning the sleeper down. Breathing can feel laboured or constricted, not because the lungs have stopped working, but because the combination of paralysis and fear tightens the subjective sense of air flow. Visual experiences vary. Some people see a shadowy figure in the doorway, a face leaning close to theirs or shapes that coil around the bed. Others report more abstract phenomena: swirling colours, flashes of light or the impression that the whole room is subtly distorted. Auditory elements are often layered on top—a low buzzing, footsteps, whispering or a voice that seems to come from just above the pillow.

Cultural narratives have long grown up around this cluster of experiences, and artists have helped give them a memorable visual form. In many European traditions, sleep paralysis is personified as an "old hag" or witch who sits on the chest and steals breath, an image echoed in Henry Fuseli's famous 1781 painting *The Nightmare*, where a squat, demonic figure crouches on a sleeping woman's torso while a ghostly horse peers from the shadows.

Modern stories of UFO abductions, in which a person describes waking frozen in bed, seeing entities by the bed or bright lights in the room, feeling probed, floated or taken through walls, often map closely onto the phenomenology of sleep paralysis, even when the experiencer interprets them in extraterrestrial rather than spiritual terms. Incubus and succubus legends—beings that immobilise sleepers and force sexual contact—can also be re-read, in many cases, as narrative frameworks wrapped around episodes of paralysis accompanied by chest pressure, genital sensations and overwhelming presence (Molendijk et al., 2017). Again, the point here is not to reduce every supernatural or abduction report to sleep physiology, but to note how a recurring pattern of bodily and perceptual events tends to be filled out with whatever explanatory resources a culture or subculture provides.

Narcolepsy presents a related but broader pattern of state instability in which hallucinations are woven into a wider tapestry of symptoms (Ahmed & Thorpy, 2010). People with narcolepsy often experience overwhelming daytime sleepiness, sudden lapses into sleep and episodes of cataplexy—brief losses of muscle tone triggered by strong emotion such as laughter or surprise. Within this context, vivid hypnagogic and hypnopompic hallucinations are common, sometimes far more frequent and elaborate than those seen in the general population. For a person with narcolepsy, slipping towards sleep on the sofa may reliably bring an intense vision of someone walking through the room, or a full-blown scene unfolding around them, even though family members nearby see nothing unusual. On awakening in the morning, they may hear voices at the bedroom door or see an intruder sit on the bed, with these episodes repeating multiple times a week rather than once in a lifetime.

In narcolepsy, REM-related processes can intrude not only at the edges of sleep but also into the middle of the day. A person may nod off briefly in a lecture, only to find that in those seconds, they have had an entire dream-like sequence, complete with voices, images and plot, which then blurs into waking reality when they lift their head. Another may experience partial paralysis while dozing in a chair, hearing people talk in the next room and seeing a figure approach, yet being unable to move until the episode clears. These are not isolated curiosities; they are part of a chronic pattern in which the boundaries between REM, NREM and wakefulness are less sharply drawn than in most people. For clinicians, the presence of frequent, vivid transition-related hallucinations alongside daytime sleepiness and cataplexy can be an important clue that narcolepsy is at work rather than a primary psychotic disorder.

Parasomnias add a further layer of complexity by showing how unusual behaviours and experiences can arise when the brain is only partially awake or partially asleep (Howell, 2012). In REM sleep behaviour disorder, for example, the usual muscle paralysis of REM fails, and the person may act out dream content—talking, flailing or even leaping from the bed in response to threats within the dream. Here, the hallucination-like content belongs to the dream itself, but its behavioural expression spills into the physical bedroom, sometimes leading to injury. Confusional arousals, often emerging from deep NREM sleep, can leave someone sitting up, talking or moving with a glazed, bewildered expression, not fully oriented to where they are or what is happening. They may mis-perceive shadows, furniture or the movements of a bed-partner, briefly treating them as threatening figures or strange creatures before sinking back into sleep.

What unites these disparate sleep disorders is not any single symptom, but a shared pattern of state disruption: REM features appearing at the wrong time, NREM arousals that stall halfway and mixtures of waking awareness with sleep-bound imagery that leave the person suspended between worlds. In such conditions, hallucinations are less an isolated phenomenon than a sign that the normal sequencing of sleep and wake has slipped out of alignment, allowing elements of one state to leak into another. The next chapter turns from these night-time misalignments to the ways in which substances can similarly disturb the brain's construction of reality, tracing how drugs and other agents open different pathways to seeing and hearing what is not there.

6

HALLUCINATIONS AND SUBSTANCES

In 1953, in a quiet room in Los Angeles, Aldous Huxley swallowed four-tenths of a gram of mescaline sulphate, sat back in an armchair and waited for the world to change. Huxley was already famous as the author of *Brave New World* and as a sharp, curious commentator on science, spirituality and culture, and he approached the drug not as a hedonist but as someone trying to observe his own mind with care. A few hours later, he would suggest that each of us is normally protected from an overwhelming flood of impressions by a mental "reducing valve" that lets through only a manageable trickle of experience. Under mescaline, he felt that valve give way. He reported in *The Doors of Perception*, "each person is at each moment capable of remembering all that has ever happened to him and of perceiving everything that is happening everywhere in the universe" (Huxley, 1954, p. 22). The folds of his trousers, the pattern on a chair, the colours of flowers in a vase seemed to expand into vast, absorbing events; time loosened, space deepened and the ordinary room around him became at once utterly familiar and strangely transformed.

Huxley's experiment is often remembered as a starting point for modern psychedelic culture, but it is also a careful reflection

DOI: 10.4324/9781003784890-7

on hallucinations and on how thin the boundary can be between "normal" perception and something more extreme. The shifting colours, moving forms and almost visionary scenes he reports are not quite everyday illusions, yet they do not look exactly like the frightening hallucinations associated with psychosis. They sit in a middle ground, as if the same perceptual system were playing in a different key. What makes his account so compelling is not just the vivid description, but the question behind it: If a small dose of a plant-derived substance can rearrange experience so profoundly, what does that say about how reality is normally put together in the mind?

This chapter uses Huxley's mescaline afternoon as a starting image, not as a standard against which all substance-related hallucinations should be measured. Many such experiences are anything but gentle or enlightening. Long-term stimulant use can give rise to the sensation of insects crawling under the skin. During severe alcohol withdrawal, people may see threatening animals, strangers or shadowy figures in the room. In delirium on a medical ward, patients can find their hospital beds transformed into battlefields, prisons or crowded trains. In other settings, hallucinations unfold within ritual and ceremony: The visions associated with ayahuasca, peyote or psilocybin may be understood as meetings with spirits, ancestors, or psychological truths rather than as "side effects". In research clinics, meanwhile, a single high-dose psychedelic session, carefully prepared and supported, is being explored as a possible turning point in depression, PTSD or addiction. Across all these situations, substances do not create hallucinations in isolation. They interact with expectations, places, life histories and cultural stories to generate worlds that feel real while they are happening.

Earlier chapters have already followed several important strands. Substances cross and connect these strands in distinctive ways. They can imitate or intensify the mechanisms described in Chapter 2—altering neuromodulators, shifting the balance between prior expectations and incoming signals—but their effects are never only about receptors and pathways. A dose of lysergic acid diethylamide (LSD) taken alone in a cramped flat after nights of poor sleep is not the same as the same dose swallowed in a quiet retreat, with therapists or guides, or on a crowded dance floor surrounded by music and strangers. The chemical is identical, yet the hallucination belongs just as much to the surrounding story, the social situation and the person's vulnerabilities as it does to the molecule itself.

Huxley's experience has therefore prompted an important question: What happens when the brain's usual "reducing valve" is pushed, chemically, into another position, and what does that reveal about hallucinations more generally? Substances provide, for better and worse, a set of rough tools for forcing open the doors of perception, and consequently, it is important to take seriously both the risks and the possibilities that arise when those doors open wider than usual, and when the worlds that appear through them cannot be neatly contained within medicine, culture or personal identity.

STYLES OF HALLUCINATION ACROSS DRUGS

Classic psychedelics such as LSD, psilocybin, mescaline and dimethyltryptamine are often what people first think of when they hear the phrase "hallucinogenic drug" (Nichols, 2004). They all act, in slightly different ways, on serotonin receptors in the cortex, as key players in how the brain builds up its model of the world. Here the focus is on what that activity feels like. Under these substances, vision usually changes first and most dramatically. Colours become unusually rich and luminous; patterns on carpets, curtains or skin seem to move, breathe or unfold into endlessly repeating shapes (Sayin, 2012). Straight lines may bend and undulate, and ordinary objects can grow halos of light or soft trails that follow their motion. With eyes closed, people often report complex internal "films": Moving geometric designs, landscapes, faces or symbolic scenes that seem to arise on their own.

These visual changes are not experienced as simple tricks like watching a poor-quality special effect. They feel layered with meaning. The brain's tendency to find patterns and complete partial information, discussed in Chapter 2 in relation to predictive processing, is pushed into the foreground, so that faint shadows on the wall become intricate forms and small coincidences in the environment seem loaded with significance. Sounds shift as well. Music may seem deeper and more detailed, as if each instrument has been separated out and then woven back together around the listener. Everyday noises—passing cars, voices in another room, the hum of a refrigerator—can take on rhythmic or symbolic qualities, sometimes momentarily becoming words or "messages" before dissolving back into ordinary sound. Body sensations change too: people may feel they are expanding, melting into their surroundings or dissolving at the edges, so that the line between "me" and "world" becomes less strict.

On the other hand, stimulant drugs like amphetamine and cocaine produce a very different kind of altered perception, especially when taken in high doses or for long periods without sleep (Parrott, 2015). At first, the world can simply feel sharpened: Lights seem brighter, sounds clearer, small movements instantly grab attention. Over time, however, this heightened alertness can tip into something more disturbing. Visual experience often becomes crowded with small, moving forms—flecks, fibres or specks on surfaces that are seen as insects, or quick flashes of movement at the edge of vision that resolve into shadowy figures. People may spend long periods scanning walls, bedding or their own skin, convinced that bugs or other contaminants are present. Tactile hallucinations are particularly common. The classic example is the sense of insects crawling on or under the skin, sometimes described as "bugs", "worms", or "glass", which can lead to intense scratching or picking.

Hearing is also affected. Someone who has been awake for days on stimulants may begin by hearing their name called or thinking they hear footsteps outside the door. As paranoia grows, these experiences often organise into more coherent but frightening sequences: Voices that seem to be commenting on them, plotting against them or discussing them in the next room. Unlike the often expansive, symbolic quality of psychedelic experiences, stimulant-related hallucinations tend to narrow the world around themes of threat and surveillance.

Dissociative drugs such as ketamine and phencyclidine add another, distinct style (Petersen et al., 2020). Instead of vivid, colourful visions or crawling insects, the dominant note is one of detachment—from the body, from the surrounding space and sometimes from time itself. These substances disrupt glutamate signalling in ways that connect back to the predictive models already discussed in Chapter 2, but they are felt most directly as changes in perspective. The room may appear to tilt, stretch or shrink; distances can feel wrong, as if the door is oddly far away or the ceiling suddenly close. Movements may leave smeared trails, and objects may appear slightly cartoon-like or flattened, but the most striking experience is often the sense of being outside oneself. People describe watching their own body from above, feeling like a spectator to their own thoughts or perceiving everything as if behind glass.

Sounds can become distorted or strangely placed. Voices in the room may seem to come from behind the head, echo in slow motion or arrive as if through a tunnel. When voice-like hallucinations occur in these contexts, they often have a mechanical, distant quality, fitting the broader impression that ordinary ownership of thoughts and perceptions has come loose. Body sensations are also profoundly altered. Limbs may feel enormous or tiny, misplaced or absent; some people feel as if they are sinking into the bed or dissolving into the floor. In contrast to the stimulant picture of hyper-alertness and persecutory detail, dissociative experiences often make the world feel unreal and the self oddly absent or duplicated, with hallucinations woven into this overall disconnection.

Nevertheless, it is important to keep in mind that not all drug-related hallucinations occur while the person is actively intoxicated. Alcohol withdrawal, sedative-hypnotic withdrawal and certain forms of drug or medication toxicity can produce delirium, where hallucinations arise within an already unstable grasp on place, time and situation. As we have already seen, in severe alcohol withdrawal, for example, the person may see small animals, insects or people moving rapidly around the room, climbing on furniture, or emerging from the walls. The scene can shift from moment to moment: An empty chair is suddenly occupied; the floor seems to swarm; the window shows a street or landscape that is not really there. These pictures are usually accompanied by confusion, agitation and rapid fluctuations in attention. Sounds may also be misheard or hallucinated—snatches of music, distant conversations, or bangs and crashes—yet, unlike the more coherent persecutory voices seen with stimulants, they tend to be fragmentary and embedded in a dream-like stream of events.

Stepping back from the individual drugs, some broad themes become visible. Psychedelics tend to exaggerate the brain's natural drive to find structure and meaning, making the constructive side of perception overt and often beautiful or uncanny. Stimulants push systems involved in salience and threat into overdrive, leading to voices, insects and hostile watchers in the environment. Dissociatives disrupt the sense of embodied, unified selfhood, producing floating viewpoints, distorted spaces and experiences in which hallucinations and radical shifts in perspective are tightly entangled.

In each case, the hallucinatory style echoes the same underlying principles introduced in Chapter 2—prediction, inference, the balancing of prior expectation against incoming evidence—but in a way that is specific to the neurochemical and physiological changes each substance brings about. At the same time, no drug ever acts on a bare brain. The same dose can yield very different worlds depending on who takes it, what they expect, where they are and what stories they already have available to make sense of unusual perceptions. Substances do not create the possibility of hallucination from nothing; rather, they tilt an already constructive perceptual system in particular directions, revealing different faces of the hallucinatory potential built into ordinary cognition.

RITUALS, RAVES AND CLINICS

Hallucinations brought on by substances rarely happen in a vacuum. They unfold in particular rooms, with particular people, under particular expectations and those surroundings shape not only what is seen and heard, but what it ends up meaning. The same vision can be welcomed as sacred, enjoyed as entertainment or feared as a sign of breakdown, depending on where and how it appears.

In many Indigenous and religious traditions, hallucinogenic plants are woven into long-standing ceremonial practices (Metzner, 1998). Ayahuasca in parts of the Amazon, peyote in Native American Church meetings, psilocybin-containing mushrooms in some Mesoamerican practices and other regional preparations are taken within carefully structured rituals led by specialists such as shamans, healers or elders. The aim is not primarily pleasure or escape, but contact with spirits, ancestors or divine forces, guidance for personal problems, or healing of illness. Within these settings, seeing animals, deities or otherworldly landscapes, or hearing spirit voices, is expected rather than surprising. Participants are prepared beforehand, guided during the experience through songs, prayers or specific procedures, and helped afterwards to interpret what happened. A terrifying jaguar might be framed as a guardian or a teacher; a painful sequence of scenes might be understood as confronting personal or collective trauma.

Accounts like those of Carlos Castaneda (1998) in *The Teachings of Don Juan: A Yaqui Way of Knowledge* helped popularise, for Western readers, a particular image of such practices—a solitary apprentice, a Native mentor and powerful plant allies that teach through visions and trials. Castaneda described encounters with entities, transformations into animals and journeys across worlds under the influence of peyote and other substances, presenting them as part of a disciplined training in "seeing". At the same time, substantial doubt has been raised about whether his fieldwork and experiences were reported as they actually occurred, with anthropologists and historians questioning key details and treating his work as at least partly fictionalised (Kostićová, 2021). His books nonetheless captured an enduring idea: that hallucinations in ritual contexts can be framed as lessons, tests or messages from non-human intelligences, rather than as meaningless by-products of intoxication.

This cultural framing has powerful effects. It can contain fear—people are told in advance that difficult material may arise, and that it has a place in a larger story. It can also assign positive value to experiences that, in another context, would be labelled simply "psychotic". At the same time, ritual spaces are not automatically safe or ideal. Unequal power between guides and participants, the commercialisation and export of sacramental plants and the mixing of traditional forms with global "psychedelic tourism" have led to well-documented problems, including exploitation and abuse (Peluso, 2014). Even so, these practices show one way in which hallucinations are made intelligible: As shared, narratively anchored events that tie individuals to communities, moral codes and cosmologies.

Recreational use tends to look very different. From the counter-cultural gatherings of the late 1960s—most famously the Woodstock rock festival—to today's clubs, raves and house parties, substances such as LSD, 3,4-Methylenedioxymethamphetamine (MDMA), ketamine, nitrous oxide and various designer drugs circulate in scenes organised around music, dancing, sex and exploration (Weir, 2000). Hallucinations in these environments often take the form of intensified sensory effects: trails on moving hands, walls "breathing", colours blooming under lights, or patterns on clothing and faces coming alive. Subculture and setting strongly shape how these changes are interpreted. Feeling merged with a crowd on a dance floor, seeing "energy" between people or experiencing music as a living presence may be taken as markers of a positive experience—sometimes even as signs of being "spiritually open" or "properly rolling". Yet the same heightened suggestibility and sensitivity to atmosphere can turn quickly. Conflict, police intervention, a bad interaction or a health scare can invert the mood, transforming connectedness into fear. People may start to feel watched or judged, hear critical or hostile voices in the noise, or perceive threatening figures in the crowd. In groups that practice harm reduction—providing water, quiet spaces, reassurance and non-judgmental support—such episodes can often be contained. In other circles, fear may be dismissed, mocked or met with encouragement to take more, deepening paranoia and confusion.

The most recent—and perhaps most debated—frontier is the clinical and quasi-clinical use of psychedelics (Garcia-Romeu et al., 2016). Leading research centres, including those at Johns Hopkins University (Griffiths & Grob, 2010) and Imperial College London (Letcher, 2024), have conducted trials in which substances like psilocybin and MDMA are administered under controlled conditions to people struggling with severe depression, PTSD, addictions or end-of-life distress. This work, popularised for general audiences by writers such as Michael Pollan, has helped bring the field into public awareness. As Pollan (2019, ch.6) notes, "the new research into psychedelics comes along at a time when mental health treatment … is so 'broken'—to use the word many psychiatrists have used in conversation with me—that the bar for approving new treatments in this area isn't terribly high".

Participants are carefully screened, meet with therapists beforehand and, during dosing sessions, often lie on a couch or bed with eyeshades and music. Afterwards, they receive guidance to process and discuss what occurred. In this setting, hallucinations are understood as potentially meaningful rather than inherently pathological. Participants may revisit traumatic memories with new emotional insight, encounter symbolic figures that express avoided truths, or feel moments of deep connection with others or the world itself. The hope is that, when properly prepared and integrated, these experiences can help loosen long-standing patterns of thought and emotion that have kept people trapped in suffering.

Parallel to these trials, a much more loosely regulated landscape has emerged: Underground therapists, spiritual guides and wellness retreats offering psychedelic sessions to paying clients. These may borrow some elements from science (screening questionnaires, talk of neuroplasticity), some from therapy (couch, tissues, "integration") and some from ritual (altars, chanting, "sacred medicine"). For many people who attend, the resulting hallucinations are described as life-changing, helping them to process grief, find new meaning or break destructive habits. Personal narratives and media coverage often emphasise dramatic positive outcomes.

Alongside these reports, however, there is growing recognition of serious controversies (Johnson et al., 2008). One set of concerns is about psychological and psychiatric risk. Even in highly controlled research settings, some participants have overwhelmingly frightening experiences, sudden resurfacing of trauma or lingering anxiety and confusion afterwards. People with vulnerability to psychosis or bipolar disorder may experience dangerous destabilisation, which is why such individuals are usually excluded from trials—yet they may still seek out underground or commercial services that do not screen carefully. There are reports of persistent perceptual changes, worsening mood or anxiety, and, more rarely, enduring psychotic symptoms after psychedelic use (Yildirim et al., 2024). This raises difficult questions about how to weigh potential benefits against possible harms, who decides what level of risk is acceptable and how long-term follow-up should be handled.

Another area of controversy concerns power, consent and ethical practice. In underground and retreat settings, those guiding sessions often hold enormous authority while being subject to little outside oversight, a dynamic made more troubling in light of historical abuses such as the CIA's MK-Ultra programme (Friesen, 2025), in which psychedelics were administered without informed consent for purposes of control and experimentation. Participants under the influence are highly suggestible and may feel dependent or indebted. There have been documented instances of sexual assault, financial exploitation and manipulation of beliefs, in which facilitators insist that particular hallucinated messages or entities confirm their own teachings or authority (Harrison et al., 2025). Even within formal trials, commentators worry about strong positive expectations—on the part of researchers, participants and media—that may shape both experience and reporting, and may make negative outcomes harder to acknowledge (Noah, 2024).

A further debate centres on how to understand the meaning of the hallucinations themselves. Are the voices, visions and felt presences encountered under psychedelics best viewed as revealing deep psychological truths, as brain-based phenomena that can nonetheless be used creatively in therapy, or as culturally patterned experiences that depend heavily on suggestion, setting and story? Proponents of psychedelic-assisted therapy argue that intense hallucinatory experiences can allow people to confront pain, shame or rigid self-images in ways ordinary conversation cannot, and that the symbolic richness of these states can open new paths for change. Critics caution that intensity is not the same as insight, and that there is a risk of treating everything seen or heard in these sessions as inherently profound. Over-interpreting hallucinated content may encourage grandiose, paranoid or magical thinking in some individuals, especially if careful integration and reality-testing are lacking. Therapists and guides must walk a narrow line between honoring people's subjective meaning and gently questioning interpretations that could fuel further distress.

RISK, VULNERABILITY AND LIFE PATHS

Substance-related hallucinations do not just punctuate isolated evenings; for many people, they mark turning points that shape how they think about themselves, their minds and their futures. Some episodes remain contained—a single intense experience that is later recalled with curiosity or ambivalence but does not fundamentally alter the course of a life. Others seem to open doors that are harder to close, contributing to longer-term problems with mood, anxiety, psychosis or substance use itself. Still others are woven into narratives of growth or awakening, even when they have been frightening.

For a substantial minority, hallucinations associated with substances remain transient. A person might have a powerful psychedelic journey in early adulthood, experience striking visuals or "entity" encounters, and then return to ordinary life without ongoing distress or impairment. The memory may become a story told to friends, an aesthetic or spiritual reference point, or simply an odd adventure. In such cases, personal and social resources—supportive relationships, stable housing and work, absence of major prior trauma or psychiatric vulnerability—often help the experience find a benign place in the life story. By contrast, when people enter altered states against a background of unresolved trauma, marginalisation or existing mental health difficulties, drug-related hallucinations can tip an already unstable balance.

Risk does not lie solely in individual biology. Social context and meaning-making play a central role in whether hallucinations become ongoing problems or sources of learning. People who have access to non-judgmental spaces to talk about what they saw and heard, who can place their experiences within frameworks that acknowledge both danger and significance, may be better able to integrate them. Others, confronted only with stigma (as "crazy") or glamorisation (as "chosen" or "enlightened"), can feel pulled towards extremes. Some may hide distressing after-effects for fear of being labelled mentally ill; others may feel pressure, from peers or inner expectations, to treat every hallucinated message as profound guidance, even when it encourages risky or isolating behaviour. Substance-induced hallucinations thus sit at the crossroads of personal vulnerability, cultural narrative and available forms of support or containment.

Over time, these experiences can become central elements of identity. A single overwhelming trip may be remembered as the moment someone "became spiritual", "saw the truth" or, conversely, "lost their mind". For people who later receive psychiatric diagnoses, early drug-related hallucinations are sometimes retrospectively reinterpreted either as the first signs of illness or as misused attempts at self-medication. For others involved in activist or spiritual communities, substance experiences and their hallucinatory content may underpin ongoing commitments and life choices. In each case, the hallucinations are not just symptoms or events; they become narrative anchors—points to which people return when explaining who they are and how they got here.

Thinking in terms of trajectories rather than isolated episodes brings this chapter into conversation with what follows. The question is no longer only what substances "do" to perception, but how people live with, remember and reinterpret those altered perceptions over months and years, and how helpers can respond. The next chapter takes up both the subjective experience of hallucinations—substance-related and otherwise—and the practical question of what can be done about them: How voices, visions and presences are felt from within; how they shape daily routines, relationships and self-understanding; and how clinicians, peers and communities try to ease distress and support more workable relationships with these experiences.

7

HALLUCINATIONS, LIVED EXPERIENCE AND TREATMENT

In the fourth century BCE, Plato (2007) closed his *The Republic* with a strange and arresting narrative, the myth of Er. A soldier, Er, the son of Armenius, is killed in battle, his body lying among the dead for ten days without decay. When he is placed on a funeral pyre, he abruptly returns to life and tells an elaborate story of what transpired while he was gone: journeys across the afterlife, judgments visited on souls, celestial mechanisms of fate and the moment when each soul chooses its next life before returning to the world. Whether read as theology, allegory or fiction, the myth of Er is a striking early exploration of a question that this chapter brings into the foreground: What happens when someone claims to have seen and heard things that others cannot, in spaces that others do not believe exist and yet insists that these experiences are as real as waking life.

Plato was not interested in diagnosing Er, but in using his story as a moral and metaphysical fable about justice, injustice and how the cosmos is ordered. From a psychological angle, though, the tale is full of features that today would prompt very different questions: a man thought to be dead describes a vivid, detailed, emotionally intense experience that seems to take place beyond ordinary perception, filled with voices, landscapes, presences and carefully

DOI: 10.4324/9781003784890-8

sequenced events, after which he returns to his community with a changed sense of reality and a new idea of how life should be lived. Plato treats this as philosophically valuable and perhaps metaphorically true, without ever asking whether Er's experience might have been a hallucination, a confabulation or the effect of a brain under extreme stress.

This gap between ancient and modern sensibilities is not simply academic. It points to a central concern: How individuals and societies live with hallucinations, and how they decide what to do with them. Er's experience could be slotted, with minimal translation, into contemporary categories such as a near-death experience (NDE), a complex vision or an extended, dream-like hallucination emerging at the border of life and death. What distinguishes these labels from Plato's original framing is not only a change in vocabulary, but a change in the kinds of questions that seem obvious to ask. Did this really happen? Was his brain hypoxic? Was this a protective illusion, a symbolic narrative or a glimpse of something beyond? Should such experiences be encouraged, treated, interpreted or explained away?

The focus now shifts from "what hallucinations are" to "how people orient themselves in relation to them, day by day". Instead of cataloguing types of voices or visual figures, the emphasis here is on lived worlds and practical choices. How does it feel to inhabit a reality in which presences appear unbidden, where the body seems to stretch, duplicate or float outside itself, or where the ordinary boundaries between self and world become porous? How do people name these experiences, conceal them, share them or weave them into their identities?

In modern settings, the question of "what to do" with experiences like Er's is where treatment enters the picture, and it is rarely a simple matter of turning hallucinations off. Just as Plato let Er's vision stand and then wove it into an ethical framework, contemporary responses range from trying to dampen or interrupt distressing experiences to helping people reinterpret and live alongside them in safer ways. Medication may reduce the intensity or frequency of voices and visions, but it can also blunt aspects of experience that the person values, creating trade-offs that have to be negotiated rather than imposed. Psychological and dialogical approaches, peer groups and community resources often focus less on erasing hallucinations and more on reshaping the relationship to them: Finding ways to question harmful commands, to set boundaries with persecutory figures or to integrate meaningful elements without being overwhelmed. As we discuss these issues, a question like "What if Er walked into a clinic today?" should hover in the background, as a reminder that treatment is not only about symptoms, but about how professionals, families and communities choose to receive someone who returns from their own unseen worlds and begins to speak.

ORIENTING TO HALLUCINATORY WORLDS

For many people who live with hallucinations, the most striking feature is not a single image, sound or presence, but the way their whole sense of reality seems to tilt. Time may stretch or compress, space may feel strangely deep or flat and the sense of self may loosen or split, as if awareness is both inside and outside the body at once.

Consider out-of-body experiences (OBEs), often described as moments when consciousness seems to drift above or beside the physical body, watching it from an external vantage point with an uncanny mixture of detachment and concern (Alvarado, 2000). In clinical settings, people recovering from surgery, birth deliveries, intensive care or acute medical crises may later report seeing themselves from above the bed, looking down on their own body and the staff working around it, as if they had briefly become spectators to their own lives.

Similar "observer" perspectives are described in some dissociative states, where a person feels detached from thoughts, feelings or bodily sensations and may picture themselves from a point near the ceiling, the doorway or a corner of the room, as though the self had stepped outside to watch what is happening. Psychologically, these episodes can be understood as an extreme form of a defence mechanism in which the mind distances itself from overwhelming fear, pain or conflict by splitting experience into a suffering body and a detached witness, trading a stable sense of unity for a fragile illusion of safety (Mitchell, 2017).

Sometimes this kind of experience takes a more specific and eerie form: Seeing a double of oneself, a doppelganger that looks identical but appears as a separate person moving through the world (Blom, 2023). People may describe catching sight of themselves sitting across the room, or feeling as if another "version" of them is standing nearby with its own mood or intention, as though their sense of self has split into two. Writers have long drawn on this image of the double, and the 18th-century Romantic writer Jean Paul's coining of the term *Doppelgänger* has become a classic literary touchstone (Webber, 1996), giving cultural shape and language to these unsettling experiences of self-duplication.

Experiences of a felt "double" are not limited to psychiatry; they also appear in extreme environments and neurological illness. Mountaineers in perilous conditions sometimes describe a mysterious "third man" climbing just ahead or beside them, offering guidance or calm, as in Ernest Shackleton's famous Antarctic expedition (McCorristine, 2014), where he and his exhausted companions reported the uncanny sense of an extra person trekking with their party. Similar companion-like figures are described by polar explorers who feel a silent presence trudging in parallel across the ice, and by neurological patients who sense someone standing just behind or next to them when no one is there, a so-called "sense of presence" that suggests the brain's maps of body, space and self can misfire in ways that conjure not only voices or visions, but an entire unseen partner at the edge of awareness.

NDEs are also relevant in this regard: People report moving through tunnels, encountering brilliant light, or meeting deceased relatives or spiritual beings, while feeling an intense clarity and peace that can make ordinary waking life seem thin by comparison (Fischer & Mitchell-Yellin, 2016). NDEs raise especially difficult questions, because they are often taken as direct evidence for life after death, yet they also show clear signatures of how the brain behaves under extreme stress. Many accounts share a family resemblance: An initial sense of leaving the body, a passage through darkness or a tunnel, encounters with intense light or with deceased relatives, a panoramic review of one's life and a moment of decision or instruction before returning. From a neuroscientific angle, there are plausible stories about such patterns that involve changes in blood flow and oxygen during cardiac arrest, waves of disinhibition in visual and temporal regions and the brain's tendency under threat to stitch fragmentary signals into a single coherent sequence—so that a brain pushed to its limits may effectively run a "last simulation", compressing memory, emotion and learned images of dying into one powerful experience (Martial et al., 2025).

These experiences also have a strong cultural footprint. Who appears at the end of the tunnel, or in the light, often reflects the person's upbringing and belief system: A Christian might encounter Jesus, Mary or angels; someone from a different religious background might meet ancestors, revered teachers or figures drawn from their own spiritual tradition; others describe more abstract presences or just an overwhelming sense of love or peace. The broad structure of NDEs may be shaped by shared human neurobiology, but the specific characters, landscapes and interpretations are usually drawn from the symbolic resources a person has available. This mix of common form and culturally inflected content makes NDEs especially interesting as examples of how brains under pressure generate experiences that feel both intensely personal and immediately meaningful.

Even if NDEs can be framed in neurocognitive terms, it remains important to approach them with respect rather than automatic debunking, and there is ongoing debate about whether they might ever provide evidence that goes beyond individual experience (Mays & Mays, 2015). For many people, an NDE is among the most significant events of their lives, reshaping values, relationships and beliefs for decades, and listening seriously does not require treating the experience as conclusive proof of an afterlife. Some researchers have tried to design ways of testing whether NDEs involve perception that cannot be explained by ordinary senses or memory: For example, by placing hidden images or symbols on high shelves or on top of equipment in resuscitation areas, visible only from a position near the ceiling and then checking whether patients who report out-of-body components can accurately describe what was there (Parnia et al., 2014). So far, such attempts have not produced clear, replicable evidence that people are seeing things from a disembodied vantage point, which strengthens the case for understanding NDEs as compelling, deeply meaningful experiences constructed by a vulnerable brain rather than as straightforward demonstrations that consciousness floats free of the body.

One important example of how hallucinatory experience intersects with ordinary life is found in grief hallucinations, sometimes described as sensory or quasi-sensory encounters with the deceased (Grimby, 1993). Large surveys suggest that between roughly a third and over half of bereaved people report some sense of the dead person's continued presence, and a substantial minority describe seeing, hearing, feeling or even smelling them, especially a deceased spouse or partner (Stokes, 2025). Many describe such encounters as deeply meaningful and even treasured, helping them sustain an emotional bond, renegotiate unfinished business and gradually absorb the reality of the loss.

In line with the earlier discussion about how to treat historical and religious testimony, it is important not to retroactively diagnose prophets, visionaries or mourners. Nevertheless, these insights about grief hallucinations place us in a better position to understand ghosts, apparitions and "visitations" from the dead as part of a recognisable human repertoire of perception—experiences that can be narrated, shared and culturally shaped, much like NDEs, without needing to appeal to supernatural mechanisms.

Alien abduction narratives provide another, very different window into how hallucinatory worlds are organised and interpreted. In the early 1960s, an American couple, Barney and Betty Hill, reported a now-famous sequence of events after driving home at night through rural New Hampshire (Bowman, 2023). They saw a strange light in the sky, noticed that time seemed to have gone missing from their journey, and later, under hypnotic regression, described being taken aboard a craft, examined by non-human beings and subjected to procedures that blended medical imagery with elements of fear, violation and cosmic significance. Whatever exactly happened that night, their account helped crystallise a template for later alien abduction stories: bright lights, paralysis or loss of bodily control, intrusive examinations, telepathic communication and a sense of being chosen or marked.

From a psychological perspective, such narratives can be understood as ways of giving shape to ambiguous bodily sensations, sleep-related phenomena (as already covered in Chapter 5) and culturally available symbols of power and otherness. As with many other experiences approached in this book, they show how hallucination-like experiences rarely arise in a vacuum; instead, they plug into existing myths, technologies and anxieties. The same core experience—waking up unable to move, sensing a presence, feeling pressure on the chest, seeing figures at the bedside—might be interpreted as a demonic attack in one era, as a visitation by ancestors in another and as alien experimentation in a culture saturated with science fiction and imagery of advanced technology.

Phantom limb experiences add yet another layer to this picture of altered worlds (Brugger, 2012). After an amputation, many people continue to feel their missing limb as vividly as before, sometimes in neutral or even comforting ways, sometimes in the form of severe pain or contorted postures that seem impossible to relieve. The brain's internal representation of the body does not instantly update when the limb is lost; instead, it continues to generate sensations as if the limb were still present.

Work by Ramachandran (1998) on body maps and phantom limbs famously showed how simple manipulations of visual feedback, such as mirror illusions, can reshape these experiences and has led to practical interventions for phantom limb pain. Mirror-box therapy and related techniques can sometimes ease phantom limb pain by giving the brain new visual feedback to reconcile with its old map, suggesting that these experiences are not simply "false signals" but the product of a negotiation between prior expectations and current sensory input. Phantom limbs highlight how deeply the sense of self is rooted in predicted bodily states. Even when sight, touch and common sense all insist that the limb is gone, the person's lived world may still include it as a stubborn, felt reality that has to be managed, worked around or slowly retrained. The body, in this sense, is not a fixed object but an ongoing construction that can lag behind physical changes, producing experiential worlds that do not quite match the shared, visible one.

Synaesthesia shows another way perception can blur, often without causing distress (Hubbard, 2007). It is estimated to occur in a minority of people (D. Johnson et al., 2013)—likely a few percent of the population—though exact figures vary depending on how strictly it is defined and how it is measured. In synaesthesia, stimulation of one sense automatically and involuntarily triggers an additional sensory experience in another. A person might hear musical notes that evoke specific colours, see letters consistently tinted or taste flavours linked to particular words. The composer Olivier Messiaen, for example, described experiencing musical chords as vivid colours (Bernard, 1986). Some synaesthetes also perceive numbers or months as fixed spatial arrangements, as if mapped around them in invisible patterns.

These experiences are usually not considered hallucinations, because synaesthetes generally know that others do not see or feel what they do, and they can tell these private sensations apart from objects in the outside world. Current research suggests that synaesthesia arises because brain areas that normally process different kinds of information (e.g., colour and shape, or sound and pitch) are more strongly connected or less clearly separated, so that activity in one system "spills over" into another and creates a secondary sensation (Cytowic & Wood, 1982). Still, synaesthesia shows how the brain can layer additional sensations on top of ordinary input, creating a personal, consistent overlay that no one else can access.

The boundary between these stable cross-sensory pairings and more disruptive hallucinations is not as sharp as diagnostic labels suggest: in both cases, the brain is generating perceptions that feel real to the person, even when they are not anchored in the shared environment.

Hypnosis offers a more controlled setting in which hallucination-like phenomena can be deliberately evoked. Under hypnotic suggestion, some people can be led to experience vivid sights, sounds or bodily sensations that are not present, or to fail to see objects that are right in front of them (Mazzoni et al., 2009). A hypnotist might suggest that the participant cannot move an arm, that a neutral stimulus is unbearably painful or that a stranger's face is unrecognisable, and the participant will report the corresponding change in experience as if it were happening automatically. These effects are not equally strong in everyone, and there is ongoing debate about what hypnosis actually is—an altered state, social role-play, focused attention or some mixture of these. Critical voices, such as Nick Spanos (1986) and others, have emphasised the importance of expectation, demand characteristics and social context, arguing that hypnotic phenomena can often be understood without positing a special trance state.

From the perspective of modern models of perception, hypnosis is especially revealing because it shows how expectations can shape, and sometimes override, what people seem to feel and see. In a hypnotic setting, when a person is strongly encouraged to believe that their arm cannot move, the brain can temporarily treat this "immobile arm" story as more trustworthy than its usual prediction that the arm is under voluntary control, so the arm really does feel stuck. A simple suggestion like "you will see a cat on the table" can tilt visual processing so that vague shadows or patterns are interpreted as a definite cat, even though nothing is actually there. In this way, hypnosis acts like a small experimental stage where beliefs, social cues and the desire to cooperate with the hypnotist can generate experiences that are, from the inside, very similar to hallucinations, even in people who have no mental disorder.

This suggestible aspect of perception also helps to make sense of how hallucination-like experiences can become partly shared, and it connects back to the wider concern, introduced at the start of the book, about how minds handle an environment saturated with powerful images and contested truths. In the same way that carefully staged videos, deepfakes and viral "evidence" can convince large groups that an event occurred exactly as shown, even when it did not, a crowd at a religious site or mass gathering can be primed to expect a miracle and be told that the sun is moving, changing colour or sending messages. Their visual systems are already leaning towards that interpretation, so individual quirks of perception—after-images, glare, fleeting distortions—are read as confirmation of the expected sign, and the reports quickly reinforce one another. Something similar can happen in collective apparitions or mass "sightings": People are not necessarily lying, but they are perceiving through a shared story that shapes what feels real to them. This makes hypnosis and related phenomena important for understanding how hallucinations can be both deeply personal and, in a looser sense, collective—rooted in individual brains, yet amplified and steered by the same social and symbolic forces that also make fake news and simulated images so convincing.

MAKING SENSE: VOICES, OTHERS AND IDENTITY

These extraordinary human experiences carry a profound immediacy for those who endure them. They confront individuals with dilemmas that unfold on several levels at once. The first challenge is ontological: What did, in fact, occur? For someone revived from cardiac arrest who recalls an intricate NDE, the vision may possess a solidity and emotional significance far deeper than ordinary waking life. Yet clinicians may reduce that same interval to a few seconds without pulse or oxygen. The experiencer must then decide: Was this a message from another realm, a neurobiological artefact or an unresolvable mystery that straddles both worlds?

A second dilemma emerges in the social sphere: whether, and to whom, to disclose. Speaking about alien abduction, visions of leaving the body, or persistent sensations from a missing limb can relieve anxiety when met with curiosity and empathy. But it can also risk disbelief, ridicule or diagnostic labelling. In institutional contexts, such disclosures may trigger psychiatric classification before understanding. Silence, by contrast, may guard against stigma while deepening isolation. Every choice carries emotional and interpersonal weight.

The third dilemma unfolds across time: How should this experience become part of one's personal story? Some individuals transform overwhelming experiences into spiritual reorientation or new identities; others struggle with lasting shame, uncertainty or vigilance. Persistent perceptual changes—such as enduring synaesthetic colours or phantom sensations—must gradually find a place in a person's sense of their own body and perception, blurring boundaries between the unusual and the normal.

Rarely do people face these perplexities without cultural scaffolding. Families, communities, media narratives and professionals all supply interpretative models. A spiritual lens might frame a NDE as a divine summons or message from ancestors, while a medical one attributes it to neurochemical misfiring or reduced oxygen supply. A trauma-centred lens interprets hallucinatory or dissociative phenomena as echoes of earlier terror and helplessness. More contemporary, technologically influenced frameworks—shaped by digital metaphors and simulation theories—see them as "system glitches" in a manipulated or virtual reality. Each lens offers something distinct: spirituality gives meaning and belonging, medicine grants a shared vocabulary and perceived legitimacy, trauma theory links present distress to historical pain, and technological metaphors express modern anxieties about control and surveillance.

This negotiation intensifies for those who hear voices. The first stage, often suffused with fear, involves confronting the perceived collapse of normality: The conviction of losing one's mind, being targeted by unseen agencies or being judged by omnipresent critics.

Voices that command, comment or insult tend to merge with a person's preexisting anxieties, reinforcing deep-seated suspicions of unworthiness or threat. Concealment is common, as people attempt to protect themselves from ridicule or institutionalisation. The realisation, "I hear voices", may itself transform self-understanding, forcing a redefinition of who one is and where one belongs.

Over time, however, many voice-hearers reconstruct meaning in ways that soften fear and restore agency. Some come to regard voices as part of the mind's internal dialogue, a collapse of boundaries between thought and sound. Others interpret them within religious frameworks—as divine messages or ancestral presences—especially when such interpretations resonate with local cultural narratives. Still others view the voices through a trauma lens, recognising in them the echoes of past abusers, internalised shame or unresolved grief. These evolving narratives do not merely modify belief; they change relationships to the voices themselves. Reframing "I am being attacked by demons" into "these voices sound like how I was spoken to as a child" transforms absolute persecution into a representation of historic pain—still painful, but no longer omnipotent.

Identity questions are interwoven throughout this meaning-making process. Many ask, "What kind of person hears voices?" In societies where hallucinations are tightly linked to mental illness or danger, dominant identity narratives evoke shame and social exclusion: "I am defective", "I am unreliable", "I am no longer one of them". Such self-descriptions subtly limit aspirations and belonging. Yet alternative communities and frameworks create space for other identities. For example, the Hearing Voices Movement—partly inspired by Julian Jaynes' theories, as discussed in Chapter 1—reframes "voice hearer" as a neutral descriptor rather than a symptom, similar to saying "I have migraines" or "I dream vividly" (Corstens et al., 2014). This approach challenges the idea that hallucinatory experiences must equal illness, gesturing instead towards diversity in human perception and consciousness.

Historically, many cultures have offered roles—such as seer, medium or healer—that validate rather than pathologise such experiences. In Indigenous traditions, auditory and visionary phenomena are often situated within communal rituals and healing practices, where they are understood as sources of guidance and communication rather than malfunction. Psychiatry can learn from these traditions—not to romanticise them, but to recognise that meaning-making frameworks already exist outside Western biomedicine that normalise and integrate anomalous experience. Building a genuinely multicultural psychology requires acknowledging that credibility, sanity and meaningfulness are not purely clinical but deeply cultural categories, shaped by power and history (Mio et al., 2023).

Community thus becomes the cornerstone of meaning-making. People who find spaces—such as Hearing Voices groups or online networks—where experiences can be described on their own terms often report relief and empowerment. In these settings, it is not agreement on explanation that matters, but the shared understanding that such experiences deserve open discussion. Voices may be spoken of as spiritual entities, fragments of consciousness or lingering traumas; what unites participants is recognition that these phenomena are real in their impact and communicable without shame. Research shows that such dialogs allow people to craft richer life narratives linking voices to personal history, relationships and social contexts rather than reducing them to pathology (Branitsky et al., 2024).

Finally, professionals and everyday listeners shape this landscape. When psychiatrists, teachers or family members respond with curiosity, ask what the voices say and validate the person's understanding, they affirm that meaning matters. When they reduce the experience to a disorder checklist, they imply the opposite—that the content and context of hallucinations are irrelevant. Families that react with panic or rigid moral judgment often drive experiences underground; those who listen without complete comprehension make disclosure less risky and the experiences more tolerable.

WORKING CLINICALLY WITH HALLUCINATIONS

Emphasising experience, culture and community does not mean that medication, medical procedures or structured therapies have no place. Some hallucinations are closely intertwined with episodes of severe illness and risk, and there is by now a substantial clinical toolkit for trying to reduce harm and restore a workable grip on shared reality. It is understandable that people may be wary of psychiatry and pharmaceuticals, not least because of the history of coercion, over-medication and the critiques raised by anti-psychiatric writers such as Szasz (2010) and Laing (1990), who pointed to the roles of power, ideology and social control in defining madness. Those critiques remain important as reminders of what can go wrong, but they do not cancel the fact that, for many, access to careful and collaborative clinical care is a crucial part of living with hallucinations rather than being overwhelmed by them.

In conditions where hallucinations appear within a psychotic picture, antipsychotic medication remains the main pharmacological tool (Sommer et al., 2012). First-generation antipsychotics such as haloperidol or fluphenazine and second-generation drugs such as risperidone, olanzapine, quetiapine, ziprasidone, aripiprazole or amisulpride can, over weeks or months, reduce the intensity and frequency of voices and other hallucinations by altering dopamine signalling in key brain pathways. For those whose hallucinations remain highly persistent despite at least two adequate trials of antipsychotics, clozapine is often considered (Nasrallah et al., 2019); its distinctive receptor profile can make it particularly helpful for treatment-resistant auditory hallucinations, though at the cost of regular blood monitoring and vigilance for rare but serious side effects such as agranulocytosis. In practice, the aim is usually to find the lowest dose that brings hallucinations into a more manageable range, rather than to eliminate every unusual perception regardless of cost, because higher doses increase the risk of weight gain, metabolic problems, movement disorders, sedation and sexual side effects.

When hallucinations arise during severe mood episodes, pharmacological choices are shaped by the underlying mood pattern as well as by the hallucinations themselves (Rothschild, 2013). In major depression with psychotic features, combinations of antidepressants and antipsychotics are common, and electroconvulsive therapy (ECT) is often recommended when voices or somatic hallucinations are accompanied by marked suicidality, stupor or refusal of food and fluid. Delivered under anaesthesia and muscle relaxation, ECT can rapidly reduce mood-congruent hallucinations and delusional guilt in ways that medication alone sometimes cannot (Salama & England, 1990).

In bipolar disorder with psychotic symptoms, mood stabilisers such as lithium, valproate or certain atypical antipsychotics (e.g., quetiapine, olanzapine or lurasidone) form the pharmacological backbone, with antipsychotic doses adjusted more aggressively during acute manic or mixed states when hallucinations are prominent (Miklowitz, 2019). Here, reducing hallucinations and stabilising mood are intertwined aims, since recurrent swings in mood increase the likelihood that voices and visions will flare again.

Hallucinations linked to neurological and medical conditions call for a different calibration of risk and benefit. We have seen that in Parkinson's disease and dementia with Lewy bodies, for example, recurring visual hallucinations of people, animals or figures in the room are common; however, many standard antipsychotics can markedly worsen motor symptoms or even provoke dangerous sensitivity reactions. Clinicians, therefore, often begin by adjusting dopaminergic Parkinson's medications, tapering or simplifying regimens in the hope that hallucinations will ease without making movement unacceptably stiff or slow. When additional medicationisnecessary,low-dosequetiapineorclozapine,orserotonin-targeting agents such as pimavanserin, may be used, with close monitoring for adverse effects (Morgante et al., 2004).

In Charles Bonnet syndrome, where complex visual scenes occur against a background of significant visual loss, detailed explanation and reassurance are usually central: Understanding that the brain is "filling in" missing visual input, and that the images do not signal psychosis or dementia, can substantially reduce distress and pharmacological treatment is generally reserved for cases where hallucinations become very intrusive or frightening.

In epilepsies with focal seizures, brief, stereotyped hallucinations—flashes of light, fragments of music, smells of burning or perfume, sudden feelings of presence—are often treated indirectly, through seizure control. Antiseizure medications such as carbamazepine, lamotrigine, levetiracetam, valproate and others are chosen according to seizure type and comorbidities (Perucca, 2005), and successful seizure management often brings a marked decrease in associated hallucinatory auras. For medically-based delirium, where vivid visual hallucinations and fluctuating confusion are common, the clinical priority is identifying and correcting the driving causes—infectious, metabolic, toxic or iatrogenic—while supporting hydration, oxygenation, orientation and sleep. Short-acting antipsychotics may be used in low doses for severe agitation or dangerous behaviour, but they are adjuncts to treating delirium, not the cornerstone.

Sleep-related hallucinations are often addressed by stabilising sleep patterns and treating specific sleep disorders. Isolated hypnagogic and hypnopompic hallucinations are usually benign; explanation, regular sleep schedules and attention to factors such as caffeine and screen use at night often suffice. When such hallucinations appear in narcolepsy, wake-promoting agents like modafinil and, in some cases, sodium oxybate for nocturnal symptoms and cataplexy may be introduced (Zhou et al., 2024). In REM sleep behaviour disorder, where people act out dreams in ways that can cause injury, low-dose clonazepam at night and environmental safety measures (removing sharp objects, padding furniture, sometimes separate beds) are standard, alongside neurological follow-up because of the condition's association with synucleinopathies such as Parkinson's disease and Lewy body dementia.

Substance-related hallucinations require yet another set of clinical tools. In alcohol withdrawal states, including delirium tremens, benzodiazepines such as diazepam, chlordiazepoxide or lorazepam are first-line to prevent seizures and calm autonomic over-activation (Grover & Ghosh, 2018); antipsychotics may be added cautiously if terrifying hallucinations contribute to agitation, but the main treatment remains adequate benzodiazepine coverage and medical support. Hallucinations emerging during stimulant intoxication with cocaine or amphetamines are treated primarily through cessation of use, quiet environments and short-term sedatives, often with temporary antipsychotics when paranoia and threatening voices are intense (Ciccarone, 2011); many episodes resolve with sustained abstinence, though a subset evolve into more chronic psychotic pictures. Hallucinations linked to classic psychedelics or dissociatives are typically approached through psychoeducation, monitoring and support for reducing or stopping use, with more formal pharmacological treatment reserved for cases that develop persistent psychosis, severe anxiety or syndromes such as hallucinogen persisting perception disorder.

Yet, it is important to emphasise that medication and medical procedures are only part of what clinical work with hallucinations involves. From the psychological side, cognitive-behavioural therapy (CBT) has been specifically adapted to address how people relate to voices and images rather than aiming to "switch them off" altogether (Haddock et al., 1998). CBT begins by developing a very detailed picture of the experiences—when they happen, what seems to trigger them, what they say or show, how the person reacts and what they believe the hallucinations can do. On that basis, the therapist and the subject identify key beliefs that fuel distress, such as "these voices are all-powerful", "they can punish my family if I disobey" or "only mad people hear voices", and then design collaborative experiments to test these beliefs in graded, safe ways. Someone might, for instance, delay or slightly modify obedience to a command while closely observing what actually happens, or systematically check whether a voice that claims to know secrets ever really produces information it could not have been inferred from context.

Alongside this, CBT works on attention and coping: learning to notice early signs that hallucinations are intensifying, using distraction or competing sounds, scheduling specific "voice time" instead of responding constantly and reducing safety behaviours—like continual checking or avoidance—that keep fear and preoccupation high. The emphasis is on changing the relationship with hallucinations so that they feel less all-controlling and the person feels more able to choose how to respond, without forcing a single "correct" explanation of what the experiences are.

Approaches influenced by the Hearing Voices Movement and trauma-informed therapies add further dimensions to this work by focusing less on getting rid of voices and more on changing the relationship with them (Higgs, 2020). Voice-focused approaches invite people to map patterns in their voices—who they sound like, when they appear, what themes they return to—and then to experiment with different kinds of dialogue: setting boundaries ("I'm not talking to you when you're shouting"), negotiating ("you can speak later, not in this meeting") or choosing to engage only with voices that feel more neutral or supportive. This can gradually shift the experience from feeling at the mercy of random, omnipotent intruders to dealing with more predictable, sometimes even partially cooperative, presences.

A widely cited example is Eleanor Longden, who has written and spoken publicly about learning, through voice-dialogue and meaning-focused work, to understand her previously terrifying voices as connected to earlier life events and unmet needs; over time, this reframing helped reduce their hostility and allowed her to study, work and build relationships while still hearing them. As Longden (2013) explains in one of her popular *Ted Talks*: "My voices were a meaningful response to traumatic life events, particularly childhood events, and as such were not my enemies but a source of insight into solvable emotional problems".

Trauma-oriented approaches start from the observation that, for many people, the tone and content of hallucinations echo earlier abuse, neglect or overwhelming fear, even when the person has not consciously made that connection. Therapy then supports the processing of those memories, traces how certain voices acquired their shaming or threatening quality, and works towards kinder narratives about the self and its survival. As links between past and present become thinkable and less overwhelming, the intensity and intrusiveness of trauma-linked hallucinations often diminish, and harsh self-judgements soften, so that these approaches complement the more symptom-focused strategies of CBT with a broader reworking of personal history and meaning.

CONCLUSION

Reality, as this book has argued, is not a neutral backdrop waiting to be registered, but something minds and cultures continually co-produce from fragmentary signals and powerful expectations. Contemporary anxieties about fake news, deepfakes and synthetic media echo, in secular form, the questions that hallucinations pose more intimately about how perception can be led astray. If images and narratives can be engineered to bypass critical scrutiny, and if brains can generate experiences that feel as solid as any event in the world, then perceptual trust becomes an achievement rather than a default. Hallucinations show how thin the boundary can be between a world that is socially shared and worlds that are privately constructed yet subjectively undeniable, without implying that reality is mere illusion. They underline that reality, as humans live it, is always mediated by bodies, histories, stories and social arrangements that decide which experiences are believed, marginalised or punished.

In this book, hallucinations have appeared as philosophical puzzles, religious encounters, clinical symptoms, early warning signs, sources of creativity and intimate companions or adversaries. Each angle highlights a common core: Experiences that feel like perception

DOI: 10.4324/9781003784890-9

despite the absence of a matching external event, drawing on sensory, emotional and narrative resources. No single explanation is sufficient, because hallucinations sit at crossroads—between expectation and sensation, memory and perception, biology and culture. What emerges is less a tidy definition than a stance: Hallucinations as rich, consequential expressions of the mind's world-building powers, sometimes painful, sometimes creative and often woven quietly into ordinary life.

The opening question—can we trust our senses?—admits neither a simple "yes" nor an unequivocal "no". As we have seen, work on predictive processing suggests that perception functions as a kind of "controlled hallucination", the brain's best guess about the causes of sensory input, constrained but never fully fixed by incoming data. When constraints weaken or expectations dominate, hallucinations appear as the loose seams of this inferential process, without implying that "anything goes" or that facts collapse into private fantasy. This view clarifies the difference between experiences anchored in a shared environment and those that drift from it, and shifts attention to the biological, psychological and social conditions that help keep perception grounded.

An integrated future psychology of hallucinations will need to keep biological, psychological and social dimensions in active conversation. Neurobiological models of predictive processing and network connectivity must remain linked to lived phenomenology, explaining not only how hallucinations arise but how they feel and unfold in daily life. Longitudinal and developmental work can show when hallucinations simply pass, when they consolidate into enduring difficulties, and how trauma, deprivation and protective relationships steer these paths. Research that follows hallucinations across psychosis, mood disorders, dissociation, neurodegeneration and substance-related states can support more mechanism-based classifications and move beyond simple symptom counting. First-person and qualitative methods are crucial to prevent hallucinations from being reduced to mere "error signals", maintaining continuity between laboratory constructs and the world people actually inhabit.

Social and technological changes introduce additional, urgent questions. Artificial intelligence can now generate images, video and voices with striking, "hallucinatory" realism and tailor them to individual vulnerabilities, externalising a form of machine hallucination into everyday information streams. This blurs boundaries between internal misperception and engineered misrepresentation, inviting doubt about both personal perception and the integrity of digital environments. Future work will need to examine how such media ecosystems interact with proneness to hallucinations and psychosis—for example, whether deepfake-rich spaces intensify persecutory ideas, or whether carefully designed virtual and augmented realities can help modulate distressing hallucinations as controlled counter-worlds. Ethical inquiry at the intersection of AI, mental health and epistemic justice will be vital, asking who controls these technologies, whose realities they amplify, and whose they silence.

A social-justice and post-colonial lens further broadens the field. Hallucinations often arise in contexts of chronic poverty, racism, displacement and violence, which shape brain development, stress physiology and interpretive frameworks, influencing who develops distressing experiences and how they are received. Psychosis risk, including hallucinations, tends to cluster in communities marked by deprivation and discrimination, indicating that prevention must include policies that reduce adversity, secure housing, and build spaces where unusual experiences can be voiced without automatic coercion. At the same time, post-colonial critiques remind us that colonial psychiatry routinely pathologised indigenous cosmologies involving visions and voice-hearing, while exporting European classifications as if they were universal. A more just psychology of hallucinations requires collaboration with communities whose healing practices—such as shamanic journeys or possession rituals—treat hallucination-like experiences as relational rather than as isolated neural malfunctions. Such partnerships can reveal alternative coping paths and expose blind spots in dominant Western models, including the tendency to individualize suffering rooted in historical dispossession and structural violence.

Taken together, these strands suggest a psychology of hallucinations that is both more modest and more ambitious. It is modest in relinquishing the search for a single master explanation, treating hallucinations instead as a family of experiences arising from overlapping mechanisms and layered meanings. It is ambitious in refusing to keep hallucinations confined to the clinic, following their implications for how societies define knowledge, allocate care and decide whose accounts of reality are taken seriously. The question "can we trust our senses?" thus gives way to a more urgent challenge: How to create worlds in which people can test and share their perceptions without shame, seek help without losing dignity, and draw on multiple traditions of understanding when experiences blur the line between the real and the imagined. Seen this way, the psychology of hallucinations becomes not a remote subspecialty, but a guide to living thoughtfully with the mind's remarkable, risky and sometimes wondrous capacity to make more than it is given.

REFERENCES

Aarsland, D., Larsen, J. P., Cummings, J. L., & Laake, K. (1999). Prevalence and clinical correlates of psychotic symptoms in Parkinson disease: A community-based study. *Archives of Neurology, 56*(5), 595–601. https://doi.org/10.1001/archneur.56.5.595

Abid, H., Ahmad, F., Lee, S. Y., Park, H. W., Im, D., Ahmad, I., & Chaudhary, S. U. (2016). A functional magnetic resonance imaging investigation of visual hallucinations in the human striate cortex. *Behavioral and Brain Functions: BBF, 12,* 31. https://doi.org/10.1186/s12993-016-0115-y

Adachi, N., & Akanuma, N. (2016). Delusions and hallucinations. In M. Mula (Ed.), *Neuropsychiatric symptoms of epilepsy* (pp. 69–89). Springer International Publishing. https://doi.org/10.1007/978-3-319-22159-5_5

Adams, R. A. (2018). Bayesian inference, predictive coding, and computational models of psychosis. In *Computational psychiatry* (pp. 175–195). Elsevier.

Ahmed, I., & Thorpy, M. (2010). Clinical features, diagnosis and treatment of narcolepsy. *Clinics in Chest Medicine, 31*(2), 371–381. https://doi.org/10.1016/j.ccm.2010.02.014

Alvarado, C. S. (2000). Out-of-body experiences. In *Varieties of anomalous experience: Examining the scientific evidence* (pp. 183–218). American Psychological Association. https://doi.org/10.1037/10371-006

Amad, A., Cachia, A., Gorwood, P., Pins, D., Delmaire, C., Rolland, B., Mondino, M., Thomas, P., & Jardri, R. (2014). The multimodal connectivity of the hippocampal complex in auditory and visual hallucinations. *Molecular Psychiatry, 19*(2), 184–191. https://doi.org/10.1038/mp.2012.181

Anderson, S. W., & Rizzo, M. (1994). Hallucinations following occipital lobe damage: The pathological activation of visual representations.

Journal of Clinical and Experimental Neuropsychology, 16(5), 651–663. https://doi.org/10.1080/01688639408402678

Association, A. P. (2022). *Diagnostic and statistical manual of mental disorders, text revision DSM-5-TR*. American Psychiatric Pub Inc.

Bartels-Velthuis, A. A., Jenner, J. A., Willige, G., van de, Os, J., van, & Wiersma, D. (2010). Prevalence and correlates of auditory vocal hallucinations in middle childhood. *The British Journal of Psychiatry, 196*(1), 41–46. https://doi.org/10.1192/bjp.bp.109.065953

Bartholomew, R. E. (2001). *Little green men, meowing nuns and head-hunting panics: A study of mass psychogenic illness and social delusion*. McFarland & Company.

Baudrillard, J. (1994). *Simulacra and simulation* (S. F. Glaser, Trans.). University of Michigan Press.

Baudrillard, J. (2009). *The gulf war did not take place* (P. Patton, Trans.). Power Publications.

Bentall, R. P. (1990). The illusion of reality: A review and integration of psychological research on hallucinations. *Psychological Bulletin, 107*(1), 82–95. https://doi.org/10.1037/0033-2909.107.1.82

Bentall, R. P., & Beck, A. T. (2004). *Madness explained: Psychosis and human nature*. Penguin.

Berkeley, G. (1982). *A treatise concerning the principles of human knowledge* (K. P. Winkler, Ed.). Hackett Publishing Company, Inc.

Bernard, J. W. (1986). Messiaen's synaesthesia: The correspondence between color and sound structure in his music. *Music Perception, 4*(1), 41–68.

Berrios, G. E. (1996). *The history of mental symptoms: Descriptive psychopathology since the nineteenth century*. Cambridge University Press.

Birchwood, M., Michail, M., Meaden, A., Tarrier, N., Lewis, S., Wykes, T., Davies, L., Dunn, G., & Peters, E. (2014). Cognitive behaviour therapy to prevent harmful compliance with command hallucinations (COMMAND): A randomised controlled trial. *The Lancet. Psychiatry, 1*(1), 23–33. https://doi.org/10.1016/S2215-0366(14)70247-0

Blom, J. D. (2023). *A dictionary of hallucinations*. Springer.

Bonnot, O., Herrera, P. M., Tordjman, S., & Walterfang, M. (2015). Secondary psychosis induced by metabolic disorders. *Frontiers in Neuroscience, 9*. https://doi.org/10.3389/fnins.2015.00177

Bowman, M. (2023). *The abduction of Betty and Barney Hill: Alien encounters, civil rights, and the new age in America*. Yale University Press.

Branitsky, A., Longden, E., Bucci, S., Morrison, A. P., & Varese, F. (2024). Group cohesion and necessary adaptations in online hearing voices Peer support groups: Qualitative study with group facilitators. *JMIR Formative Research, 8*, e51694. https://doi.org/10.2196/51694

Brugger, P. (2012). Phantom limb, phantom body, phantom self: A phenomenology of "Body hallucinations." In J. D. Blom & I. E. C. Sommer

(Eds.), *Hallucinations: Research and practice* (pp. 203–218). Springer. https://doi. org/10.1007/978-1-4614-0959-5_16

Calabrese, J., & Khalili, Y. A. (2023). Psychosis. In *StatPearls [internet]*. StatPearls Publishing. https://www.ncbi.nlm.nih.gov/sites/books/NBK546579/

Cassidy, C. M., Balsam, P. D., Weinstein, J. J., Rosengard, R. J., Slifstein, M., Daw, N. D., Abi-Dargham, A., & Horga, G. (2018). A perceptual inference mechanism for hallucinations linked to striatal dopamine. *Current Biology*, 28(4), 503–514.e4. https://doi.org/10.1016/j.cub.2017.12.059

Castaneda, C. (1998). *The teachings of Don Juan: A Yaqui way of knowledge.* University of California Press.

Castor, H. (2015). *Joan of Arc: A history.* Harper Perennial.

Cavanna, A. E., Trimble, M., Cinti, F., & Monaco, F. (2007). The "bicameral mind" 30 years on: A critical reappraisal of Julian Jaynes' hypothesis. *Functional Neurology*, 22(1), 11.

Cheyne, J. A. (2003). Sleep paralysis and the structure of waking-nightmare hallucinations. *Dreaming*, 13(3), 163–179. https://doi.org/10.1023/A: 1025373412722

Ciccarone, D. (2011). Stimulant abuse: Pharmacology, cocaine, methamphetamine, treatment, attempts at pharmacotherapy. *Primary Care*, 38(1), 41–58. https://doi.org/10.1016/j.pop.2010.11.004

Corstens, D., Longden, E., McCarthy-Jones, S., Waddingham, R., & Thomas, N. (2014). Emerging perspectives from the hearing voices movement: Implications for research and practice. *Schizophrenia Bulletin*, 40(Suppl_4), S285–S294. https://doi.org/10.1093/schbul/sbu007

Cowan, J. D. (2015). Geometric visual hallucinations and the structure of the visual cortex. In *The neuroscience of visual hallucinations* (pp. 217–253). John Wiley & Sons, Ltd. https://doi.org/10.1002/9781118892794.ch10

Ćurčić-Blake, B., Ford, J. M., Hubl, D., Orlov, N. D., Sommer, I. E., Waters, F., Allen, P., Jardri, R., Woodruff, P. W., David, O., Mulert, C., Woodward, T. S., & Aleman, A. (2017). Interaction of language, auditory and memory brain networks in auditory verbal hallucinations. *Progress in Neurobiology*, 148, 1–20. https://doi.org/10.1016/j.pneurobio.2016.11.002

Cytowic, R. E., & Wood, F. B. (1982). Synesthesia: I. A review of major theories and their brain basis. *Brain and Cognition*, 1(1), 23–35.

D'Agostino, A., & Limosani, I. (2010). Hypnagogic hallucinations and sleep paralysis. In M. Goswami, S. R. Pandi-Perumal, & M. J. Thorpy (Eds.), *Narcolepsy: A clinical guide* (pp. 87–97). Springer. https://doi.org/10.1007/978-1-4419-0854-4_8

de Leede-Smith, S., & Barkus, E. (2013). A comprehensive review of auditory verbal hallucinations: Lifetime prevalence, correlates and mechanisms in healthy and clinical individuals. *Frontiers in Human Neuroscience*, 7, 367. https:// doi.org/10.3389/fnhum.2013.00367

Descartes, R. (1984). *The philosophical writings of Descartes* (Vol. 2; J. Cottingham, R. Stoothoff, & D. Murdoch, Trans.). Cambridge University Press.

Draaisma, D. (2009). *Disturbances of the mind* (B. Fasting, Trans.). Cambridge University Press.

Eck, D. (1998). *Darsan: Seeing the divine image in India.* Columbia University Press.

Fénelon, G. (2013). Hallucinations associated with neurological disorders and sensory loss. In R. Jardri, A. Cachia, P. Thomas, & D. Pins (Eds.), *The neuroscience of hallucinations* (pp. 59–83). Springer. https://doi.org/10.1007/978-1-4614-4121-2_4

Fénelon, G., & Alves, G. (2010). Epidemiology of psychosis in Parkinson's disease. *Journal of the Neurological Sciences, 289*(1), 12–17. https://doi.org/10.1016/j.jns.2009.08.014

Fénelon, G., Mahieux, F., Huon, R., & Ziégler, M. (2000). Hallucinations in Parkinson's disease: Prevalence, phenomenology and risk factors. *Brain, 123*(4), 733–745. https://doi.org/10.1093/brain/123.4.733

Ffytche, D. H. (2008). The hodology of hallucinations. *Cortex, 44*(8), 1067–1083. https://doi.org/10.1016/j.cortex.2008.04.005

Fischer, J. M., & Mitchell-Yellin, B. (2016). *Near-death experiences: Understanding visions of the afterlife.* Oxford University Press.

Fletcher, P. C. (2017). Predictive coding and hallucinations: A question of balance: Comment on powers, mathys, and corlett (2017) "Pavlovian conditioning-induced hallucinations result from overweighting of perceptual priors. *Cognitive Neuropsychiatry, 22*(6), 453–460. https://doi.org/10.1080/13546805.2017.1391083

Ford, J. M., Palzes, V. A., Roach, B. J., Potkin, S. G., van Erp, T. G. M., Turner, J. A., Mueller, B. A., Calhoun, V. D., Voyvodic, J., Belger, A., Bustillo, J., Vaidya, J. G., Preda, A., McEwen, S. C., & Mathalon, D. H. Functional Imaging Biomedical Informatics Research Network (2015). Visual hallucinations are associated with hyperconnectivity between the amygdala and visual cortex in people with a diagnosis of schizophrenia. *Schizophrenia Bulletin, 41*(1), 223–232. https://doi.org/10.1093/schbul/sbu031

Freud, S. (2014). *Psycho-analytic notes on an autobiographical account of a case of paranoia.* White Press.

Friedman, J. H. (1991). The management of the levodopa psychoses. *Clinical Neuropharmacology, 14*(4), 283.

Friesen, P. (2025). The ghosts of psychedelic science: Haunting and moral repair. *Neuroethics, 19*(1), 2. https://doi.org/10.1007/s12152-025-09622-4

Friston, K. J. (2005). Hallucinations and perceptual inference. *Behavioral and Brain Sciences, 28*(6), 764–766. https://doi.org/10.1017/S0140525X05290131

Frith, C. (1996). The role of the prefrontal cortex in self-consciousness: The case of auditory hallucinations. *Philosophical Transactions of the Royal Society B: Biological Sciences, 351*(1346), 1505–1512. https://doi.org/10.1098/rstb.1996.0136

Fusar-Poli, P., De Pablo, G. S., Rajkumar, R. P., López-Díaz, Á, Malhotra, S., Heckers, S., Lawrie, S. M., & Pillmann, F. (2022). Diagnosis, prognosis, and treatment of brief psychotic episodes: A review and research agenda. *The Lancet Psychiatry, 9*(1), 72–83.

Garcia-Romeu, A., Kersgaard, B., & Addy, P. H. (2016). Clinical applications of hallucinogens: A review. *Experimental and Clinical Psychopharmacology, 24*(4), 229–268. https://doi.org/10.1037/pha0000084

Gregory, R. L. (1980). Perceptions as hypotheses. *Philosophical Transactions of the Royal Society of London. B, Biological Sciences, 290*(1038), 181–197. https://doi.org/10.1098/rstb.1980.0090

Griffiths, R. R., & Grob, C. S. (2010). Hallucinogens as medicine. *Scientific American, 303*(6), 76–79.

Grimby, A. (1993). Bereavement among elderly people: Grief reactions, post-bereavement hallucinations and quality of life. *Acta Psychiatrica Scandinavica, 87*(1), 72–80. https://doi.org/10.1111/j.1600-0447.1993.tb03332.x

Grover, S., & Ghosh, A. (2018). Delirium tremens: Assessment and management. *Journal of Clinical and Experimental Hepatology, 8*(4), 460–470. https://doi.org/10.1016/j.jceh.2018.04.012

Haddock, G., Tarrier, N., Spaulding, W., Yusupoff, L., Kinney, C., & McCarthy, E. (1998). Individual cognitive-behavior therapy in the treatment of hallucinations and delusions: A review. *Clinical Psychology Review, 18*(7), 821–838. https://doi.org/10.1016/S0272-7358(98)00007-5

Hall, R. J., Meagher, D. J., & MacLullich, A. M. J. (2012). Delirium detection and monitoring outside the ICU. *Best Practice & Research Clinical Anaesthesiology, 26*(3), 367–383. https://doi.org/10.1016/j.bpa.2012.07.002

Harrison, T. R., Faber, S. C., Zare, M., Fontaine, M., & Williams, M. T. (2025). Wolves among sheep: Sexual violations in psychedelic-assisted therapy. *The American Journal of Bioethics: AJOB, 25*(1), 40–55. https://doi.org/10.1080/15265161.2024.2433423

Hartl, E., Gonzalez-Victores, J. A., Rémi, J., Schankin, C. J., & Noachtar, S. (2017). Visual auras in epilepsy and migraine—An analysis of clinical characteristics. *Headache, 57*(6), 908–916. https://doi.org/10.1111/head.13113

Harvey, P. D., & Walker, E. (2013). *Positive and negative symptoms in psychosis: Description, research, and future directions.* Routledge.

Hersh, K., & Borum, R. (1998). Command hallucinations, compliance, and risk assessment. *The Journal of the American Academy of Psychiatry and the Law, 26*(3), 353–359.

Higgs, R. N. (2020). Reconceptualizing psychosis. *Health and Human Rights, 22*(1), 133–144.

Hobson, J. A. (2009). REM sleep and dreaming: Towards a theory of protoconsciousness. *Nature Reviews Neuroscience, 10*(11), 803–813. https://doi.org/10.1038/nrn2716

Hoffman, R. E., & Hampson, M. (2012). Functional connectivity studies of patients with auditory verbal hallucinations. *Frontiers in Human Neuroscience*, 6. https://doi.org/10.3389/fnhum.2012.00006

Hohwy, J. (2025). A metaphysics for predictive processing. *Synthese*, 206(2), 87. https://doi.org/10.1007/s11229-025-05169-2

Howell, M. J. (2012). Parasomnias: An updated review. *Neurotherapeutics*, 9(4), 753–775. https://doi.org/10.1007/s13311-012-0143-8

Hubbard, E. M. (2007). Neurophysiology of synesthesia. *Current Psychiatry Reports*, 9(3), 193–199. https://doi.org/10.1007/s11920-007-0018-6

Huxley, A. (1954). *The doors of perception*. Perennial.

Jaballah, F., Romdhane, I., Nasri, J., Ferhi, M., Bellazrag, N., Saidi, Y., & Mannaii, J. (2022). Focal epilepsy and psychosis symptoms: A case report and review of the literature. *Annals of Medicine and Surgery*, 84, 104862.

Jaynes, J. (2000). *The origin of consciousness in the breakdown of the bicameral mind*. Mariner Books.

Johnson, D., Allison, C., & Baron-Cohen, S. (2013). The prevalence of synesthesia. *Oxford Handbook of Synesthesia*, 1, 3–22.

Johnson, M., Richards, W., & Griffiths, R. (2008). Human hallucinogen research: Guidelines for safety. *Journal of Psychopharmacology*, 22(6), 603–620. https://doi.org/10.1177/0269881108093587

Johnson, M. K. (1997). Identifying the origin of mental experience. In *The mythomanias*. Psychology Press.

Karnouskos, S. (2020). Artificial intelligence in digital media: The era of deepfakes. *IEEE Transactions on Technology and Society*, 1(3), 138–147. https://doi.org/10.1109/TTS.2020.3001312

Kasper, B. S., Kasper, E. M., Pauli, E., & Stefan, H. (2010). Phenomenology of hallucinations, illusions, and delusions as part of seizure semiology. *Epilepsy & Behavior*, 18(1), 13–23. https://doi.org/10.1016/j.yebeh.2010.03.006

Kelson, M., Santos, T., Athanasios, A., & Fitzsimmons, A. (2022). Out of sight, am I losing my mind? A case report on visual release hallucinations – Charles bonnet syndrome. *Psychiatry Research Case Reports*, 1(2), 100036. https://doi.org/10.1016/j.psycr.2022.100036

Khaled, S. M., Brederoo, S. G., Yehya, A., Alabdulla, M., Woodruff, P. W., & Sommer, I. E. C. (2023). Cross-cultural differences in hallucinations: A comparison between middle Eastern and European community-based samples. *Schizophrenia Bulletin*, 49(Supplement_1), S13–S24. https://doi.org/10.1093/schbul/sbac086

Kostićová, Z. M. (2021). *From Academic Anthropology to Esoteric Religion*. https://doi.org/10.1163/15700593-20211005

Laing, R. D. (1990). *The divided self: An existential study in sanity and madness*. Penguin Books.

Lakshminarasimhan, K., Buck, J., Kellendonk, C., & Horga, G. (2025). A corticostriatal learning mechanism linking excess striatal dopamine and auditory hallucinations. *bioRxiv*, 2025.03.18.643990. https://doi.org/10.1101/2025.03.18.643990

Le Bon, O. (2020). Relationships between REM and NREM in the NREM-REM sleep cycle: A review on competing concepts. *Sleep Medicine, 70*, 6–16. https://doi.org/10.1016/j.sleep.2020.02.004

Letcher, A. (2024). Psychedelia Britannia: Druids on drugs. In *Modern religious druidry: Studies in paganism, Celtic identity, and nature spirituality* (pp. 97–119). Springer.

Linscott, R. J., & Os, J. (2013). An updated and conservative systematic review and meta-analysis of epidemiological evidence on psychotic experiences in children and adults: On the pathway from proneness to persistence to dimensional expression across mental disorders. *Psychological Medicine, 43*(6), 1133–1149. https://doi.org/10.1017/S0033291712001626

Linszen, M. M. J., de Boer, J. N., Schutte, M. J. L., Begemann, M. J. H., de Vries, J., Koops, S., Blom, R. E., Bohlken, M. M., Heringa, S. M., Blom, J. D., & Sommer, I. E. C. (2022). Occurrence and phenomenology of hallucinations in the general population: A large online survey. *Schizophrenia (Heidelberg, Germany), 8*(1), 41. https://doi.org/10.1038/s41537-022-00229-9

Loftus, E. F. (1993). The reality of repressed memories. *American Psychologist, 48*(5), 518–537. https://doi.org/10.1037/0003-066X.48.5.518

Longden, E. (2013). *The Voices in My Head* [Video recording]. https://www.ted.com/talks/eleanor_longden_the_voices_in_my_head

Luhrmann, T. M., Padmavati, R., Tharoor, H., & Osei, A. (2015). Differences in voice-hearing experiences of people with psychosis in the U.S.A., India and Ghana: Interview-based study. *The British Journal of Psychiatry, 206*(1), 41–44. https://doi.org/10.1192/bjp.bp.113.139048

Lyndon, S., & Corlett, P. R. (2020). Hallucinations in post-traumatic stress disorder: Insights from predictive coding. *Journal of Abnormal Psychology, 129*(6), 534–543. https://doi.org/10.1037/abn0000531

Lysaker, P. H., Pattison, M. L., Leonhardt, B. L., Phelps, S., & Vohs, J. L. (2018). Insight in schizophrenia spectrum disorders: Relationship with behavior, mood and perceived quality of life, underlying causes and emerging treatments. *World Psychiatry, 17*(1), 12–23. https://doi.org/10.1002/wps.20508

Malhi, G. S., Green, M., Fagiolini, A., Peselow, E. D., & Kumari, V. (2008). Schizoaffective disorder: Diagnostic issues and future recommendations. *Bipolar Disorders, 10*(1p2), 215–230. https://doi.org/10.1111/j.1399-5618.2007.00564.x

Martial, C., Fritz, P., Gosseries, O., Bonhomme, V., Kondziella, D., Nelson, K., & Lejeune, N. (2025). A neuroscientific model of near-death experiences. *Nature Reviews Neurology, 21*(6), 297–311. https://doi.org/10.1038/s41582-025-01072-z

Mays, R. G., & Mays, S. B. (2015). Explaining near-death experiences: Physical or non-physical causation? *Journal of Near-Death Studies, 33*(3), 125.

Mazzoni, G., Rotriquenz, E., Carvalho, C., Vannucci, M., Roberts, K., & Kirsch, I. (2009). Suggested visual hallucinations in and out of hypnosis. *Consciousness and Cognition, 18*(2), 494–499. https://doi.org/10.1016/j.concog.2009.02.002

McCarthy-Jones, S., Smailes, D., Corvin, A., Gill, M., Morris, D. W., Dinan, T. G., Murphy, K. C., Anthony O'Neill, F., Waddington, J. L., Australian Schizophrenia Research Bank, Donohoe, G., & Dudley, R. (2017). Occurrence and co-occurrence of hallucinations by modality in schizophrenia-spectrum disorders. *Psychiatry Research, 252,* 154–160. https://doi.org/10.1016/j.psychres.2017.01.102

McCorristine, S. (2014). Polar otherworlds: Dreams and ghosts in arctic exploration. *Nimrod: The Journal of the Ernest Shackleton Autumn School, 8,* 86–101.

McCutcheon, R., Beck, K., Jauhar, S., & Howes, O. D. (2018). Defining the locus of dopaminergic dysfunction in schizophrenia: A meta-analysis and test of the mesolimbic hypothesis. *Schizophrenia Bulletin, 44*(6), 1301–1311. https://doi.org/10.1093/schbul/sbx180

Metzner, R. (1998). Hallucinogenic drugs and plants in psychotherapy and shamanism. *Journal of Psychoactive Drugs, 30*(4), 333–341. https://doi.org/10.1080/02791072.1998.10399709

Miklowitz, D. J. (2019). *The bipolar disorder survival guide: What you and your family need to know.* The Guilford Press.

Mio, J. S., Barker, L. A., Rodríguez, M. M. D., & Gonzalez, J. (2023). *Multicultural psychology.* Oxford University Press.

Mitchell, J. L. (2017). *Out-of-body experiences: A handbook.* Crossroad Press.

Molendijk, M. L., Montagne, H., Bouachmir, O., Alper, Z., Bervoets, J.-P., & Blom, J. D. (2017). Prevalence rates of the incubus phenomenon: A systematic review and meta-analysis. *Frontiers in Psychiatry, 8.* https://doi.org/10.3389/fpsyt.2017.00253

Morgante, L., Epifanio, A., Spina, E., Zappia, M., Di Rosa, A. E., Marconi, R., Basile, G., Di Raimondo, G., La Spina, P., & Quattrone, A. (2004). Quetiapine and clozapine in Parkinsonian patients with dopaminergic psychosis. *Clinical Neuropharmacology, 27*(4), 153. https://doi.org/10.1097/01.wnf.0000136891.17006.ec

Munro, A. (2006). *Delusional disorder: Paranoia and related illnesses.* Cambridge University Press.

Nasar, S. (2011). *A beautiful mind.* Simon & Schuster.

Nasrallah, H. A., Fedora, R., & Morton, R. (2019). Successful treatment of clozapine-nonresponsive refractory hallucinations and delusions with pimavanserin, a serotonin 5HT-2A receptor inverse agonist. *Schizophrenia Research, 208,* 217–220. https://doi.org/10.1016/j.schres.2019.02.018

Nichols, D. E. (2004). Hallucinogens. *Pharmacology & Therapeutics, 101*(2), 131–181. https://doi.org/10.1016/j.pharmthera.2003.11.002

Nichols, M. D. (2019). *Malleable Mara: Transformations of a Buddhist symbol of evil.* SUNY Press.

Noah, S. (2024, April 4). How Psychedelic Clinical Trials Might Be Susceptible to Expectation. *UC Berkeley Center for the Science of Psychedelics.* https://psychedelics.berkeley.edu/how-psychedelic-clinical-trials-might-be-susceptible-to-expectation/

Ohayon, M. M., Priest, R. G., Caulet, M., & Guilleminault, C. (1996). Hypnagogic and hypnopompic hallucinations: Pathological phenomena? *The British Journal of Psychiatry,* 169(4), 459–467. https://doi.org/10.1192/bjp.169.4.459

Onofrj, M., Russo, M., Delli Pizzi, S., De Gregorio, D., Inserra, A., Gobbi, G., & Sensi, S. L. (2023). The central role of the thalamus in psychosis, lessons from neurodegenerative diseases and psychedelics. *Translational Psychiatry,* 13(1), 384. https://doi.org/10.1038/s41398-023-02691-0

Onofrj, M., Taylor, J. P., Monaco, D., Franciotti, R., Anzellotti, F., Bonanni, L., Onofrj, V., & Thomas, A. (2013). Visual hallucinations in PD and Lewy body dementias: Old and new hypotheses. *Behavioural Neurology,* 27(4), 703924. https://doi.org/10.3233/BEN-129022

Ostwald, P. F. (1985). *Schumann: The inner voices of a musical genius.* UPNE.

Parkinson, J. (1817). *An essay on the shaking palsy.* Whittingham & Rowland.

Parnia, S., Spearpoint, K., de Vos, G., Fenwick, P., Goldberg, D., Yang, J., Zhu, J., Baker, K., Killingback, H., McLean, P., Wood, M., Zafari, A. M., Dickert, N., Beisteiner, R., Sterz, F., Berger, M., Warlow, C., Bullock, S., Lovett, S., & Schoenfeld, E. R. (2014). AWARE—AWAreness during REsuscitation—A prospective study. *Resuscitation,* 85(12), 1799–1805. https://doi.org/10.1016/j.resuscitation.2014.09.004

Parrott, A. C. (2015). Why all stimulant drugs are damaging to recreational users: An empirical overview and psychobiological explanation. *Human Psychopharmacology: Clinical and Experimental,* 30(4), 213–224. https://doi.org/10.1002/hup.2468

Peluso, D. (2014). *Ayahuasca shamanism in the Amazon and beyond.* In B. Caiuby Labate & C. Cavnar (Eds.), *Ayahuasca's attractions and distractions: Examining sexual seduction in shaman-participant interactions* (pp. 231–255). Oxford University Press.

Perucca, E. (2005). An introduction to antiepileptic drugs. *Epilepsia,* 46(s4), 31–37. https://doi.org/10.1111/j.1528-1167.2005.463007.x

Petersen, M., Garg, U., & Ketha, H. (2020). Hallucinogens—Psychedelics and dissociative drugs. In H. Ketha & U. Garg (Eds.), *Toxicology cases for the clinical and forensic laboratory* (pp. 295–303). Elsevier.

Plato, & Lane, M. (2007). *The Republic* (D. Lee, Trans.). Penguin Classics.

Pollan, M. (2019). *How to change your mind: What the new science of psychedelics teaches us about consciousness, dying, addiction, depression, and transcendence.* Penguin Books.

Porter, R. (1987). *A social history of madness: Stories of the insane.* Weidenfeld & Nicolson.

Ramachandran, V. S., & Hirstein, W. (1998). The perception of phantom limbs. The d. O. Hebb lecture. *Brain,* 121(9), 1603–1630. https://doi.org/10.1093/brain/121.9.1603

Riahi, I. (2014). Ancient minds not conscious. *Zeitschrift Für Junge Religionswissenschaft*, 9. https://doi.org/10.4000/zjr.222

Rollins, C. P. E., Garrison, J. R., Simons, J. S., Rowe, J. B., O'Callaghan, C., Murray, G. K., & Suckling, J. (2019). Meta-analytic evidence for the plurality of mechanisms in transdiagnostic structural MRI studies of hallucination status. *eClinicalMedicine*, 8, 57–71. https://doi.org/10.1016/j.eclinm.2019.01.012

Rothschild, A. J. (2013). Challenges in the treatment of major depressive disorder with psychotic features. *Schizophrenia Bulletin*, 39(4), 787–796. https://doi.org/10.1093/schbul/sbt046

Sacks, O. (2013). *Hallucinations*. Vintage.

Saks, E. R. (2007). *The center cannot hold: My journey through madness*. Grand Central Publishing.

Salama, A. A. A., & England, R. D. (1990). A case study: Schizophrenia and tactile hallucinations, treated with electroconvulsive therapy. *The Canadian Journal of Psychiatry*, 35(1), 86–87. https://doi.org/10.1177/070674379003500116

Sayin, Ü. (2012). A comparative review of the neuro-psychopharmacology of hallucinogen-induced altered States of consciousness: The uniqueness of some hallucinogens. *NeuroQuantology*, 10(2).

Schott, G. D. (2007). Exploring the visual hallucinations of migraine aura: The tacit contribution of illustration. *Brain*, 130(6), 1690–1703. https://doi.org/10.1093/brain/awl348

Schreber, D. P., & Dinnage, R. (2000). *Memoirs of my nervous illness*. New York Review Books.

Scull, A. (2015). *Madness in civilization: A cultural history of insanity, from the bible to freud, from the madhouse to modern medicine*. Princeton University Press.

Sedley, W., Gander, P. E., Kumar, S., Kovach, C. K., Oya, H., Kawasaki, H., Howard, M. A. III, & Griffiths, T. D. (2016). Neural signatures of perceptual inference. *eLife*, 5, e11476. https://doi.org/10.7554/eLife.11476

Seneviratne, U. (2010). Fyodor Dostoevsky and his *falling sickness*: A critical analysis of seizure semiology. *Epilepsy & Behavior*, 18(4), 424–430. https://doi.org/10.1016/j.yebeh.2010.05.004

Seth, A. (2021). *Being you: A new science of consciousness*. Dutton.

Shevlin, M., Dorahy, M., & Adamson, G. (2007). Childhood traumas and hallucinations: An analysis of the national comorbidity survey. *Journal of Psychiatric Research*, 41(3–4), 222–228. https://doi.org/10.1016/j.jpsychires.2006.03.004

Shives, L. R. (2007). *Basic concepts of psychiatric-mental health nursing*. Lippincott Williams & Wilkins.

Sirriyeh, E. (2015). *Dreams and visions in the world of Islam: A history of Muslim dreaming and foreknowing*. I.B. Tauris.

Sluhovsky, M. (2007). *Believe not every spirit: Possession, mysticism, & discernment in early modern Catholicism*. University of Chicago Press.

Smith, D. B. (2007). *Muses, madmen, and prophets: Hearing voices and the borders of sanity.* Penguin Books.

Sommer, I. E., Daalman, K., Rietkerk, T., Diederen, K. M., Bakker, S., Wijkstra, J., & Boks, M. P. M. (2010). Healthy individuals with auditory verbal hallucinations; Who are they? Psychiatric assessments of a selected sample of 103 subjects. *Schizophrenia Bulletin, 36*(3), 633–641. https://doi.org/10.1093/schbul/sbn130

Sommer, I. E. C., Slotema, C. W., Daskalakis, Z. J., Derks, E. M., Blom, J. D., & van der Gaag, M. (2012). The treatment of hallucinations in schizophrenia spectrum disorders. *Schizophrenia Bulletin, 38*(4), 704–714. https://doi.org/10.1093/schbul/sbs034

Spanos, N. P. (1986). Hypnotic behavior: A social-psychological interpretation of amnesia, analgesia, and "trance logic. *Behavioral and Brain Sciences, 9*(3), 449–467. https://doi.org/10.1017/S0140525X00046537

Sprevak, M., & Smith, R. (2023). An introduction to predictive processing models of perception and decision-making. *Topics in Cognitive Science.* https://doi.org/10.1111/tops.12704

Stephensen, H. (2025). Double alienation: A phenomenological perspective on psychosis. *Phenomenology and the Cognitive Sciences,* 1–21.

Sterzer, P., Adams, R. A., Fletcher, P., Frith, C., Lawrie, S. M., Muckli, L., Petrovic, P., Uhlhaas, P., Voss, M., & Corlett, P. R. (2018). The predictive coding account of psychosis. *Biological Psychiatry, 84*(9), 634–643. https://doi.org/10.1016/j.biopsych.2018.05.015

Stokes, P. (2025). Sensing presence: Deathbots and bereavement hallucination. *Phenomenology and the Cognitive Sciences.* https://doi.org/10.1007/s11097-025-10064-9

Strakowski, S. M. (1994). Diagnostic validity of schizophreniform disorder. *The American Journal of Psychiatry, 151*(6), 815–824. https://doi.org/10.1176/ajp.151.6.815

Szasz, T. S. (2010). *The myth of mental illness: Foundations of a theory of personal conduct.* Harper Perennial.

Tachibana, M., Inada, T., Ichida, M., & Ozaki, N. (2021). Factors affecting hallucinations in patients with delirium. *Scientific Reports, 11*(1), 13005. https://doi.org/10.1038/s41598-021-92578-1

Tart, C. (2000). *States of consciousness.* iUniverse.

Telles-Correia, D., Moreira, A. L., & Gonçalves, J. S. (2015). Hallucinations and related concepts—their conceptual background. *Frontiers in Psychology, 6.* https://doi.org/10.3389/fpsyg.2015.00991

Toh, W. L., Thomas, N., Robertson, M., & Rossell, S. L. (2020). Characteristics of non-clinical hallucinations: A mixed-methods analysis of auditory, visual, tactile and olfactory hallucinations in a primary voice-hearing cohort. *Psychiatry Research, 289,* 112987. https://doi.org/10.1016/j.psychres.2020.112987

Van Der Kolk, B. A. (1998). Trauma and memory. *Psychiatry and Clinical Neurosciences*, 52(S1), S52–S64. https://doi.org/10.1046/j.1440-1819.1998.0520s5S97.x

Waters, F., Blom, J. D., Dang-Vu, T. T., Cheyne, A. J., Alderson-Day, B., Woodruff, P., & Collerton, D. (2016). What is the link between hallucinations, dreams, and Hypnagogic–Hypnopompic experiences? *Schizophrenia Bulletin*, 42(5), 1098–1109. https://doi.org/10.1093/schbul/sbw076

Waters, F., Ling, I., Azimi, S., & Blom, J. D. (2024). Sleep-related hallucinations. *Sleep Medicine Clinics*, 19(1), 143–157. https://doi.org/10.1016/j.jsmc.2023.10.008

Webber, A. J. (1996). *The Doppelgänger: Double visions in German literature*. Clarendon Press.

Weir, E. (2000). Raves: A review of the culture, the drugs and the prevention of harm. *CMAJ*, 162(13), 1843–1848.

Wible, C. G., Preus, A. P., & Hashimoto, R. (2009). A cognitive neuroscience view of schizophrenic symptoms: Abnormal activation of a system for social perception and communication. *Brain Imaging and Behavior*, 3(1), 85–110. https://doi.org/10.1007/s11682-008-9052-1

Wood, M. (2004). *The road to Delphi: The life and afterlife of oracles*. Picador.

Wright, N. T. (Ed.). (2008). *The resurrection of the son of God*. Fortress Press.

Yates, K., Lång, U., Peters, E. M., Wigman, J. T. W., McNicholas, F., Cannon, M., DeVylder, J., Ramsay, H., Oh, H., & Kelleher, I. (2021). Hallucinations in the general population across the adult lifespan: Prevalence and psychopathologic significance. *The British Journal of Psychiatry*, 219(6), 652–658. https://doi.org/10.1192/bjp.2021.100

Yildirim, B., Sahin, S. S., Gee, A., Jauhar, S., Rucker, J., Salgado-Pineda, P., Pomarol-Clotet, E., & McKenna, P. (2024). Adverse psychiatric effects of psychedelic drugs: A systematic review of case reports. *Psychological Medicine*, 54(15), 4035–4047. https://doi.org/10.1017/S0033291724002496

Zeman, A. (2002). *Consciousness: A user's guide*. Yale University Press.

Zhou, X., Chen, J., Xu, B., & Chen, L. (2024). Evaluation of pitolisant, sodium oxybate, solriamfetol, and modafinil for the management of narcolepsy: A retrospective analysis of the FAERS database. *Frontiers in Pharmacology*, 15. https://doi.org/10.3389/fphar.2024.1415918

Zhuangzi (2003). *Zhuangzi: Basic writings*. Columbia University Press.

Zmigrod, L., Garrison, J. R., Carr, J., & Simons, J. S. (2016). The neural mechanisms of hallucinations: A quantitative meta-analysis of neuroimaging studies. *Neuroscience and Biobehavioral Reviews*, 69, 113–123. https://doi.org/10.1016/j.neubiorev.2016.05.037

INDEX

For Product Safety Concerns and Information please contact our EU
representative GPSR@taylorandfrancis.com
Taylor & Francis Verlag GmbH, Kaufingerstraße 24, 80331 München, Germany